TOPICS
IN
GERONTOLOGY

TOPICS
IN
GERONTOLOGY

Selected Annotated Bibliographies

Edited by
Thomas O. Blank

Bibliographies and Indexes in Gerontology, Number 22

Greenwood Press
Westport, Connecticut • London

Library of Congress Cataloging-in-Publication Data

Topics in gerontology : selected annotated bibliographies / edited by
   Thomas O. Blank.
      p. cm.—(Bibliographies and indexes in gerontology, ISSN
   0743-7560 ; no. 22.)
      Includes indexes.
      ISBN 0-313-28337-0 (alk. paper)
      1. Gerontology—Bibliography. I. Blank, Thomas O., 1947- .
   II. Series.
   Z7164.O4T66   1993
   [HQ1061]
   016.6126′7—dc20   93-9311

British Library Cataloguing in Publication Data is available.

Library of Congress Catalog Card Number: 93-9311
ISBN: 0-313-28337-0
ISSN: 0743-7560

First published in 1993

Greenwood Press, 88 Post Road West, Westport, CT 06881
An imprint of Greenwood Publishing Group, Inc.

Printed in the United States of America

The paper used in this book complies with the
Permanent Paper Standard issued by the National
Information Standards Organization (Z39.48-1984).

10 9 8 7 6 5 4 3 2 1

CONTENTS

PREFACE

The tremendous growth in gerontology in the last few decades has made it imperative that professionals and those training to be professionals in research, teaching, and service related to aging and old age be able to specialize and yet to see their own "piece" of the field in relation to other areas of aging-related work. The plethora of narrowly-defined monographs and bibliographies, on the one hand, and general textbooks on the other, must be supplemented with innovative vehicles for considering gerontology in both its depth of research and breadth of interest.

The goal in writing this book is be innovative in responding to that need. The authors aim to give to students and professionals a set of essays and annotated bibliographies that individually provide in-depth explorations of specific areas of gerontology and together comprise an introduction to the richness and expanse of aging-related research and theory. Unlike most other books in gerontology, it is not limited to one perspective or one level of interest, but includes aspects of psychology, sociology, health care, anthropology, and biological sciences.

Like the book's concept, the authorship is innovative. The book arose from a requirement for participation in a Graduate Research Fellowship Program in Gerontology at the Travelers Center on Aging of the University of Connecticut. The Travelers Center is a public-private partnership of the Travelers Insurance Companies and the University of Connecticut to conduct research and training to better the lives of older persons in Connecticut and throughout the nation. With funding from the Provost's Office of the University and administration through the Social and Behavioral Sciences Division of the Travelers Center on Aging and the School of Family Studies, each year since 1987 a selected group of graduate students in a range of disciplines at the University of Connecticut at Storrs has been awarded research fellowships in gerontology. As Fellows, they conduct a major individual or collaborative project and participate in an intensive year-long seminar.

During the 1990-1991 academic year, the Fellows completed two bibliographies related to their research focus as part of their participation in the seminar. One of the bibliographies was to be in their own area of interest and expertise, whereas the second was to be complementary in topic but from a distinctly different disciplinary perspective from their own.

The group of fellows included two Ph. D. candidates in family studies, one of whom is trained in nursing, a Ph. D. candidate in nutrition, and master's degree students in nursing and biobehavioral sciences. Thus, the range of interests and resultant bibliographies is broad. One former Fellow who recently completed a Ph. D. in family studies on the history of gerontology, is contributing a bibliography in this area. The instructor for the seminar, who is Division Director of the Social and Behavioral Sciences Division of the Travelers Center and a faculty member in Family Studies, served as editor of the bibliographies and contributed the introductory essay.

Readers from many areas of the wide field of gerontology should find bibliographies that directly bear upon their interests, and all gerontology students and professionals can catch a few glimpses of aspects of gerontology that they seldom explore. All told, this volume reflects (and, we hope, expands) the scope of the exciting domain of developing and applying a growing understanding of the mechanisms and physiological, psychological, social, and societal effects of aging in the latter part of the 20th century.

FORMAT AND APPROACH IN THE BIBLIOGRAPHIES

Unlike virtually all texts and readers, this volume will address not only social gerontology, or only physiological and biological aspects, or only practice issues. Instead, attention will be addressed to social, behavioral, and biological aspects of aging in specific bibliographies, and consideration will be given in critiques that address value for both researchers and practitioners.

Each chapter is devoted to detailed consideration of a specialized topic within the broad field of gerontology. Every effort was made to include "stops" at a number of places along the road map of gerontology representing some of the major disciplines and orientations discussed in the Introduction. Several of the topics have been primarily explored in experimental research, others by qualitative means. Some are very micro-level in focus; while others are at a larger-scale place in the topology of gerontology. The order of chapters follows the road from more macro-level, societal aspects of gerontology progressively to more micro-level topics explored using more experimental, quantitative approaches.

Each chapter begins with a brief essay providing the reader with a guide to the "state of the art" on that topic. Each bibliographic entry includes a full citation for the article, chapter, or book, a clear description of its contents and main findings or main themes, and a brief critique of the value of the reference. The emphasis has been placed on recent articles, although "classics" in each field are included to give the reader a feeling for the history of that topic within gerontology.

Beginning with the history of gerontology as a discipline, the social science chapters move to areas of family relationships, decision-making about health care, policy issues about termination of life-sustaining technologies, and conclude with a pair of chapters that examine rituals about death and dying, but from very different perspectives. The second portion of the book turns toward more physiological processes related to aging from the relatively macro-level examination of sleep disorders and drug use to a chapter that includes both social and biological studies of Alzheimer's Disease, concluding with micro-level topics concerned with chemistry and hormonal changes.

Readers can probably best begin by reading the introductory essay and the introduction to each chapter to get an idea of the coverage. They can then begin with the chapter or chapters closest to their own fields and spread out from there to topics with which they are less familiar. Alternatively, they can begin with a detailed consideration of a topic and use the subject index to lead them into specific citations in various chapters that deal with that topic. In either case, the chapters taken together form a picture of the breadth and expanse of gerontology and taken separately provide a compilation of current knowledge on a set of specialized topics.

ACKNOWLEDGMENTS

The editor and the authors gratefully acknowledge the support of the Vice President and Provost of the University of Connecticut, Thomas Tighe, for the Travelers Center on Aging activities on the campus, a large part of which has been directed to the fellowship program. Also, Lucille Nahemow originated the fellowship program while she was Associate Director of the Campus Branch of the Travelers Center. Her foresight in developing the program (and her use of a more general annotated bibliography as a component of the course) has enabled us to develop these bibliographies. Caroline Garside deserves our gratitude for preparation of the indexes. We also are grateful to George F. Butler, Acquisitions Editor at Greenwood, for his support of this unique project and Maureen Melino, Coordinating Editor, for her guidance through the process of preparing the manuscript.

Finally, as Editor I wish to express my thanks to the fellowship students, who began these bibliographies as a course requirement, but did such a good job that I could not let them end there. In spite of changing personal situations, they have persevered through drafts and revisions (including evaluations of each other's work) to make their bibliographies complete, up-to-date, and of maximum usefulness.

INTRODUCTION: THE FIELD OF GERONTOLOGY AND THE BIBLIOGRAPHIES

Thomas O. Blank

Since the beginning of this century, the size of the elderly population of this country-- and across the world-- has grown faster than any other part of the population. In the coming decades, that growth will accelerate, until by 2020 fully one out of five Americans (more than one out of four adults) will be over the age of 65. The single fastest growing age group is those over 85; by 2020 there will be four times as many very old persons as there are today. For the first time in history, every person born (at least in industrialized societies) is likely to grow old-- to end up in the "old person" category-- before he or she dies.

The rapid increase in both absolute numbers and percentage of the elderly population has led to an explosion of interest in scientific investigations of aging. No major organizations in gerontology existed until the beginnings of the Gerontological Society in 1945. Now, not only are there several scientific and practitioner organizations both within the United States and internationally, but the AARP, American Association of Retired Persons, is the single largest membership organization in the country, with over 30,000,000 members.

On the one hand, many current issues in gerontology focus on changes with the aging process that may be problematic, such as physiological changes in virtually all systems of the body, resulting in changing, usually declining, ability to relate effectively to environmental demands, and reduction in roles available to people as both they and society grow older. On the other hand, they also include a growing interest in the ways older persons-- and society-- respond successfully and positively to their later years.

These interests clearly range from the personal level of changes in the needs, capabilities, and activities of persons as they grow old to the societal one of the ways these changes affect the rest of society. In turn, the societal issues are expressed both in a national debate about whether or not older persons are receiving too high a proportion of social service spending in the country and at the smaller scale of the relationships between older persons and younger members of their families. It is especially important to understand the relationship of elderly to family as the nature of the family changes with fewer children, a high level of divorce, and families with both married partners in the work force as the norm.

The explosion of popular and research interest is reflected in an accelerating trend in training needs. The Association for Gerontology in Higher Education (1991) lists over 900 institutions of higher learning in the U.S. offering at least one gerontology course; there are over 300 post-baccalaureate programs. Formal programs in gerontology are offered in community colleges and universities, and there are now two Ph. D. programs. There are also many certificate programs at both graduate and undergraduate levels that may be taken separately from a degree program. The proliferation of programs, often offered by faculty with little or no training in gerontology themselves, requires instructional and reference materials suitable for use in the broad spectrum of programs available.

As knowledge in gerontology continues to increase at a rapid rate, there is a danger that individual practitioners, faculty, and students become increasingly compartmentalized, focusing on a very narrow band of specialized interests. Articles, monographs, and even many texts reflect this narrowing of interest at the individual level. An alternative to such compartmentalization is found in the range of basic texts, which regularly try to cover all areas of knowledge. Given all the publications in gerontology and the huge number of areas of interest in this multi-disciplinary field, the most that can be accomplished in such texts is a cursory glance at each of the hundreds of topics.

Unlike virtually all texts and other educational materials, this volume does not address only social gerontology, or only physiological and biological aspects, or only practice issues. Instead, attention is given to social, behavioral, and biological aspects of aging in specific bibliographies, while the critiques of specific items indicate value for both researchers and practitioners.

This book uses an innovative approach that combines a collection of carefully annotated bibliographies on a sampling of topics across the broad spectrum of gerontology with "road maps" to the field in the form of brief essays about each topic. This introductory chapter includes several components: 1) a description of the range of interests to be found in gerontology, 2) definition and discussion of some core concepts and methods of gerontology, 3) brief overviews of a number of topics that are of interest to gerontologists today, 4) a guide to journals and handbooks of importance to those interested in gerontology as a scholarly area of interest and as a professional approach to practice in many disciplines, and 5) a description of the approach used in each bibliographic chapter.

WHAT IS GERONTOLOGY?

Coming from the Greek roots of *gerontos*--old man-- and *logos*--knowledge about or study of-- gerontology is basically the study of old people. In fact, though, it includes the study of two quite different aspects of "oldness": the state of old age and the process of aging. That is, gerontologists are concerned both with what it is like to *be* old and how people *get there* through the process of aging. In the first case, gerontologists study age groups as categories of persons, comparing one group to another. In the latter case, they focus more directly on the temporal process that begins at some point well before one is old and ends when that person (or animal) dies in old age. Although the ways to approach these two studies are quite distinct, they are united in a focus on time which is much more obvious and central to gerontology than to many other areas of scientific study and theory. Categories of age reflect, among other things, the influence of time-- how long someone has been alive and how much experience he or she has had, the residue of time and its cumulative effects. Process studies are interested in both how time changes someone and how some aspects of the person or other organism remain stable in spite of the passage of time.

The exploration of age, not surprisingly, is very complex. The need to pay attention to time is one aspect of this complexity, but so is the fact that both the category of being old and the process of growing old are a combination of biological, social, psychological, situational, and other forces that are pulled apart and treated as though they have separate effects at great risk of distortion. Because of this, gerontology has developed as a multidisciplinary enterprise; no one discipline is felt to have a sufficient range of perspective or methods to do an adequate job of understanding old age or the processes of aging. We will look more fully at the implications of the multidisciplinary nature of gerontology shortly.

One danger in defining gerontology as the study of (old) age and aging is that it does not give adequate attention to the fact that being and becoming old can only be understood within the context of being young and coming of age. An old truism talks about aging as a process that begins at birth, but often gerontology defines aging as something that only occurs to old people (or makes them old). Instead, old age is best seen in the context of the lifespan of each individual and the context of the social/historical conditions in which individuals age.

Terms and Concepts

Before proceeding, it is important to compare and contrast several pairs of basic terms.

Age and Aging. An important distinction underlying much of the preceding discussion is that between age and aging. "Age" is a reference to a category, a placement based on time. "Aging," on the other hand, is the process of moving through time,-- moving, if you will, from age to age. In turn, each of these is a complicated package of factors, not a simple word with a single definition.

Gerontologists agree that age, by itself, is not an explanation of anything. Rather, it is an index of something (many somethings) else. For example, age is an index of a certain amount of experience, of a set of social roles that are given to people on the basis of their age, of physical maturation, and of a self-perception (for example, as "over the hill" or "getting better every day"). Much of the research of gerontology is concerned with looking at older people as a group, to see if they do things differently from other groups, if they have different roles, if they have different needs than other age groups. An important issue in today's society is the fact that the age group we categorize as elderly is getting so much bigger than it has ever been; this has grave implications about what roles people of different ages should play and how much service should be directed to people specifically because of their age.

Individuals can be classified into age categories in several ways. The crudest, most obvious-- and thus, most used-- is **chronological age**. The way to know whether someone is old is simply to know how long it has been since that person was born. This tells us very little about whether that person is like other old persons and different from younger ones. It is, of course, the way that age is measured for access to an array of government services and age-based offers. A more precise approach to age, but unfortunately a much more difficult one to measure and use in everyday life, is **functional age**. Functional age focuses on how the person performs along one or more important dimensions, such as physical performance or cognitive acuity. A classic example of functional age at the younger end of the age range is intelligence testing. In this case, the functional age of a child is defined by comparing his or her responses to the average level of responses at different ages to obtain a ratio which tells whether the child is "younger," "older," or the same functional age in comparison to his or her chronological age. A concrete example of the greater value of functional age than chronological age in at least some situations is the statement by one of President Reagan's doctors after he was shot in 1982. Although he was 70, the doctor stated that Reagan had the organ systems of a 40-year old, and that his functional age in that regard was what saved his life.

"Aging," as already noted, is more a movement through time rather than a placement within it. Aging is a process. At the level of the individual, aging is a matter of ontogenesis, intra-individual change through the life span. Aging is the growth, transformation, and sometimes decline of a system as the individual moves along the temporal dimension. Of course, the "system" may be the whole person or biological, social, functional, or other aspects. When we put large numbers of people together and compare them in terms of aging, we are looking for the inter-individual variations in how people change through time. For example, we may be interested in the aging process as it usually occurs in men compared to its usual process over time in women.

Related to the differentiation between age and aging is a parallel distinction between age differences and age changes. Age differences are the differences shown when age groups or age categories are compared to each other at a point in time, whereas age changes or more properly the processes of aging, the reflection of the movement through time.

Gerontology and geriatrics. The focus of this book is on gerontology. As already defined, this is the study of old age and aging. Geriatrics, on the other hand, is the medical treatment of people in later life, especially as they experience diseases that may accompany aging. Geriatrics is, thus, limited to treatment; researchers within the medical and clinical sciences are gerontologists, and their research results are part of gerontology. That will be clearly seen in several of the chapters to follow.

Underlying Dimensions or Themes of Gerontology

As is already apparent, gerontology is composed of a wide variety of facets and foci. Gerontologists study age categories and aging processes; they may look at small-scale phenomena or large-scale ones. Several dimensions underlie the enterprise of gerontology, dimensions on which we can place specific studies and specific uses of gerontological knowledge. Together, these dimensions can help us to describe a topological space or map of gerontology. For convenience these dimensions will be described as though they are dichotomies, but it is important to realize that many, if not most, specific expressions of gerontology are combinations or mixtures of characteristics from both extreme poles of the dimensions:

1. Macro-level vs. micro-level. Gerontologists can focus on very large scale (macro-) aspects of aging or on very small-scale (micro-) ones. Examples of the macro-scale end of the dimension are studies of the demography of age, that is, the distribution of age categories in space or studies of the way social status is stratified by age, whereas examples of micro-scale studies are ones that focus on individuals or even down to the level of individual cells. The range from macro-level to micro-level within gerontology is extraordinarily large in comparison to other fields of study.

2. Societal vs. individual. Related to the macro-micro distinction is one between approaches that are concerned with individual motivations or needs and those that are concerned with, for example, the implications for society of increasing percentages of older persons. Societal gerontology is concerned with

how the social structure works, whereas individual approaches may be focused on a wide range of individual factors, from biology to psychology.

3. <u>Change vs. stability</u>. Many studies of gerontology are done precisely so that change can be revealed. Many theories, too, emphasize that change is an inevitable result of aging. Various models, however, conceptualize change in very different ways. For example, stage theorists (such as Erikson in terms of personality) hypothesize that all people change in systematic ways over time by moving through a series of qualitatively different phases. On the other hand, many non-stage-oriented theorists stress that change is the result of reactions to external forces that may or may not be universal across persons; some of these additionally conceive of aging as a process of deterioration in functioning from some earlier, higher level. On the other hand, other researchers and theorists try to discover the continuities or stabilities across time; personality theorists like McCrae and Costa (1990), for example, feel that the continuities in certain sorts of traits outweigh and overshadow the changes brought about by changing physiology or psychological outlook or, for that matter, changing social and environmental conditions.

4. <u>Active/optimistic vs. passive/pessimistic</u>. Related to change and stability are a pair of dimensions that concern the degree to which aging is seen as a matter for optimism, especially if an active organism able to have effects on both its environment and itself is posited as a part of later life. Some theories and types of research reveal the role of activity and self-expression among elderly, and these tend to portray quite an optimistic picture of the potential for growth in later life. Others emphasize a more passive view of older persons as under the control of forces-- either outside themselves, such as social stereotypes, or internal biological changes-- that make them what they are and can be. Although there is no necessary reason why such an approach would be negative or pessimistic (for example, society could have very positive stereotypes about aging or biological changes could be for the better), often passive-oriented concepts of aging are quite pessimistic.

5. <u>Basic/scientific vs. applied/practitioner</u>. A final dimension places gerontologists in a quite different way. Although the term gerontology is often defined as "the scientific study of aging and old age," there are two things wrong with this definition. First, a growing contingent of gerontological researchers do not think of themselves as scientists but as humanists; they study aging "systematically" but not "scientifically," at least not in the sense most people use that term. Second, gerontology is really a blend of both research and practice. That is, there are many gerontologists who do not do research but who apply the fruits of that research to providing a wide array of services to older persons (and sometimes their families); these services range from financial assistance to physical therapy, from nursing to senior center programs, and from assistance to older persons in their own homes to nursing home administration. Gerontology is based on a strong pair of beliefs that only by grounding practice

in the best knowledge base derived from research can practice be most effective and that the development of systematic knowledge requires a constant interaction with the ways that knowledge may be applied.

Doing gerontology, then, by necessity, is a matter of being involved in a larger network of ways of approaching aging and old age. Of course, any researcher or practitioner is located somewhere in this space, not everywhere. Any activity can only focus on a small piece of the bigger picture. While specialization is necessary to further the goals of gerontology, when specialization is not informed by at least an appreciation of the work and findings of others in gerontology-- and even in lifespan studies-- is likely to be distorted and lopsided. The result is that such efforts are less useful and effective than they might otherwise be.

The chart on the following pages places some of the disciplines that are part of the gerontological undertaking into a two-dimensional space. Those with a more basic scientific disciplines are on the top and applied ones on the bottom of the pages. Further, they range from micro-level disciplines on the left to macro-level ones on the right. Of course, many other dimensions can also be used to organize the disciplines, often cutting across the dimensions used here. The figure is titled "Branches of the 'Tree' Feeding into Gerontology," but in fact most of these many disciplines and approaches have developed quite independently from one another. Part of the problem of the gerontologist-- and the challenge-- is the lack of a "trunk" to provide the structure for these many branches to relate clearly to each other.

A PRIMER ON METHODS

When gerontologists wish to develop or use systematic information, they will use methods as tools to gather and analyze their data. The goals of all research are to describe, explain, or modify the ways people think, act, or experience their worlds. The goals of gerontologists are to do so concerning the process of aging and the effects of being old. Ultimately, they are trying to solve a puzzle about the influence of age and aging. A full discussion of methods in gerontology is beyond the scope of this chapter. It is important, however, that readers of the bibliographies are aware of the rudiments of gerontological research to be able to get the greatest benefit from the annotations. The broad canvas of gerontology, not surprisingly, requires a breadth of methods. Thus, brief discussions of data-gathering approaches and data-analytic techniques will be helpful.

BRANCHES OF THE "TREE"

Biology   Genetics   Chemistry   Physics   Psychology

Biochemistry   Biomechanics

"Basic Science"

Nutritional Science   Kinesiology

Communications

Micro-
*level*_____

Nursing   Dietetics   Pharmacy   Clinical Psychology

[Geriatrics]

Medical Technology   Physical Therapy

"Applied Science"

Occupational Therapy

Speech and Hearing

Counselling

Recreation, Exercise, and Leisure

FEEDING INTO GERONTOLOGY

Sociology   Political Science   Economics   Anthropology   Humanities
(Cross-cultural)

Geography   History
(Cross-time)

"Basic Science"

Demography   Policy Analysis

Social Psychology

Macro-
level
_____

Social Work   Planning   Public Policy

Law   Arts

"Applied Science"

Architecture and Design

Health Care Systems Administration

How Gerontologists Gather their Data

Like the field itself, the varied methods gerontologists use to gather data can be categorized on several important dimensions. At its root, data-gathering follows one of two broad approaches: asking questions or observing activity. In turn, one can ask questions in many ways of many sources, and one can observe activity ranging from large social rituals to chemical reactions.

One dimension it is useful to consider is an open/closed dimension. If we take asking questions as one approach, then we can place various ways of asking questions on a continuum that ranges from very open to very closed. Open questioning is exemplified by an interview in which a person is simply asked to tell his or her life story, without specific prompting about what to include. Indeed, one may ask questions without even being present, as when a researcher studies diaries or novels and looks for themes. Scales, in which the older person is presented with a specific set of questions and can answer them using only a "yes" or a "no," is on the other end of the continuum. Between these extremes are many variations-- interviews in which a person is asked a specific set of questions but allowed to answer in any way he or she pleases, scales that give specific stimuli but allow the person to give various types and length of answers, archival studies in which hospital records are coded and categorized, and so on. Similarly, observations of activity can range from simply observing people or animals in their natural environments and recording whatever happens in some way to placing people in very restrictive, artificial laboratory situations, giving them very specific stimuli, and observing a very limited range of responses (such as happens in a reaction time study when a light comes on and the person pushes a button as quickly as possible).

In experimental designs independent variables are carefully introduced to participants (or into tissue or other samples in a very micro-level, biological study) in a controlled way and then specific dependent variables are measured and analyzed in a precise way. For many, this approach is the epitome of scientific research. Experiments are of necessity on the closed end of the dimension. While many gerontologists use an experimental approach, it is important to remember that experimental designs are but one way of gathering the data necessary for sound gerontological research.

The open or closed approaches to data-gathering often are differentiated as qualitative and quantitative research; however, the latter differentiation strictly speaking has to do with the way data are analyzed, not the way they were gathered. Thus, there are mixed cases, for example, when data that were gathered in open interviews are subsequently reduced to a small number of categories and analyzed in a quantitative, statistical analysis. Rather than dealing with the nuances of data analysis (interested readers can refer to a book by Baltes, Reese, and Nesselroade, 1977, or chapters in almost all texts for further detail on these issues), we will turn to a brief consideration of the way time and change, the primary interests of gerontological research, are represented in several time sampling designs used by gerontologists.

Time Sampling and the Age/Period/Cohort Problem

Some gerontologists are interested only in specifying how a group of older persons acts or thinks. These researchers find their old age sample and then describe it in a detailed way. Although this is an important and very useful way to study age and aging, it does not provide the kind of information that can be used to examine and compare competing interpretations or explanations of why that group acts or thinks as it does.

The vast majority of research done by gerontologists interested in comparative explanations is done at one point in time, using a cross-sectional design. In this design, several age groups are compared to each other on whatever variables are of interest to the researcher. This approach is sufficient if the goal of research is to define the characteristics of various age groups as category factors. In other words, it can reveal age differences. It is not, however, a very adequate way of getting at exactly what many gerontologists are interested in--the process of aging and age changes that occur as people go through that process.

There are several reasons for this. Foremost is the obvious one-- to know how something proceeds through time it is essential to <u>look</u> through time. A longitudinal design that follows a process over time is the basic starting point for understanding process. However, even a longitudinal design is no guarantee that differences revealed in a study are truly age changes. To understand this, we must understand the significance of three concepts-- age, period, and cohort. All three are historical or temporal factors, but the histories they present to the researcher are quite distinct from each other.

Age, or maturation, is the composite of the processes of aging as they are expressed in an individual. It is the focus of concern for many gerontologists, but by no means all of them, and it is intertwined with several other constellations of factors whenever one does gerontological research.

Every research study is done at some time or set of times, and this boundness of findings to specific times of testing is called a *period effect*. That is, if I study retirement adjustment by doing a questionnaire study in 1992, all I am really finding is how people retiring in 1992 deal with retirement. Since the meaning of retirement has been changing over time and is likely to continue to do so, I am making a leap of faith when I assert that what I find in my current study is, in fact, what adjustment to retirement is all about; those who retire in 1992 may be unusual in some way and, thus, not representative of how people retire at other times (not to mention other places!).

The third factor is *cohort*. A cohort is simply a group that comes into a system at the same time. When gerontologists use chronological age as the basis for categorizing people into age groups, they are usually interested in birth cohorts; that is, in groups of people born at about the same time. Another cohort factor is represented for all of us who have attended college and become members of the "Class of 19xx." A particular cohort moves through time in tandem, more or less as a unit. Cohort membership, in turn, is merely an index for many variations by time of entry into life or into old age. These include any characteristics of the whole population that are systematically different in different cohorts, such as education level or degree of religiosity. They also include the combination of major events that have occurred during the lifetimes of groups of persons and the ages those people were when those events occurred.

For example, the birth cohorts of 1900 and 1920 (and 1940 to some degree) had vivid experiences of the Great Depression and the Second World War, while birth cohorts of 1960 and 1980 did not. In this way, all of those prior to the mid-1940's differ from the cohorts that were born after those events. Yet, the three "older" cohorts differ from each other in the timing of those events in relation to their own aging process. The Great Depression and the Second World War came well after entry into adulthood for the cohort of 1900 and at time of the earliest memories for the cohort of 1940. The cohort of 1920, however, experienced both of these events as they moved into young adulthood. Their lives were in many ways the most touched of all by the events: they grew up as relative prosperity turned into economic upheaval, and they (the males at least) were the ones who went to war. Glen Elder (1974) persuasively has argued how those specific events, coming when they did, set apart the cohorts around 1920 from those who came before and those who came after. A similar case could be made for many other major events, ranging from other military conflicts (for example, the Vietnam War or the Gulf incursion) to natural disasters to more positive events like the landing on the moon.

Each of these three factors can be thought of in a static way. In this case, age is personal "make-up" at a point in time, period the environmental situation at a point in time, and cohort is location in age structure at that point in time. Alternatively, each can be seen as a dynamic process-- age as psychosocial and biological unfolding, period as a progression of historical events, and cohort as a group marching through time together (often referred to as cohort flow). Whether seen in a static or dynamic way, the fact that age, period, and cohort are intertwined even though they derive from different sources produces one of the key problems of interpretation in gerontology.

Consider a typical cross-sectional design. The researcher gathers data that enable him to compare the ways older persons do something-- let us say, perform on an intelligence test-- to the ways younger ones do that same thing. If differences are found, the researcher would like to say they are the result of age changes. Can he or she say that? Unfortunately not with a great deal of confidence, because the cross-sectional design presents problems deriving from both cohort and period. First of all, period is not even considered in such a time sample; it is simply ignored (or "held constant," if one wants to use a less pejorative term). Cohort, on the other hand, is completely confounded with age; the two cannot be separated. Every 60 year old comes from the birth cohort of 1932, while every 20 year old is in the cohort of 1972. Thus, any differences that are found are: 1) the result not of age as such but of an interwoven blend of age and cohort, and 2) only representative of the one period in which the data were gathered. Cross-sectional designs can only be used to examine true age-maturational effects when neither cohort nor period have any significant effects; of course, that is a rare state of affairs at best.

A longitudinal design does a far better job of separating age and cohort, but a price is paid for that "unconfounding." In a longitudinal design, age is varied across different periods of time, but in most cases only one cohort is examined. Thus, cohort is controlled only by being treated as though it has no effect, while period and age are as confounded in this design as age and cohort are in a cross-sectional one.

Other designs are possible, as is a combination of several (see Schaie's 1965 General Developmental Model). There has been considerable debate in gerontology as to whether any of the designs or combinations is truly effective, but for most purposes, the question is moot; almost all research is done using cross-sectional designs because others are much too expensive and present too many practical problems about time, including change over time in the meaning of measures, in the composition of samples, etc. (see Baltes, Reese, & Nesselroade, 1977, for a good overview of methodological issues).

Given the methodological problems of measurement, analysis, and the interplay of age, cohort, and period effects in time sampling, clarity about research goals and about the limitations of particular methods are both important. All the problems do *not* mean that a particular study or type of study is valueless, but they do mean that great care must be taken in interpretation to keep from going beyond what the data really are able to show. Not every method is problematic for attaining every goal; what is essential is to be able to approximate a good "fit" between methods and goals. From the point of view of a researcher, the likelihood of such a fit should determine choice of methods. From the vantage point of a consumer of research, a knowledge of the strengths and limitations of various methods in relation to specific research goals can be a guide to evaluation of the quality and utility of a particular set of findings.

For example, if a research goal is to describe how older people respond to artificial tasks in comparison to young, then a cross-sectional study observing narrowly-defined behavioral choices in a laboratory setting (a very closed approach to observation) is appropriate and useful. If one's research goal is to explore how people's approach to decision-making changes over time, however, that same study might be quite useless. Instead, one should make a longitudinal examination of more naturalistic decisions, either by observing behaviors in settings appropriate across ages (for example, shopping) or by asking people to describe their own decision-making processes. In other words, research is always a matter of imperfect choices, but those choices are best made and the results of the research best interpreted knowing full well the limitations and faults of what was chosen (and the different but also problematic limitations and faults inherent in the non-chosen alternatives).

THE HISTORY OF GERONTOLOGY IN BRIEF

Although the first bibliographic chapter focuses on sources to explore the history of gerontology, several aspects of that history are so essential for consideration of the research and theory themes that have dominated gerontology that a very brief history at this point will provide a necessary foundation. Early in this chapter, it was noted that only since World War Two has there been a major thrust toward systematic studies of age and aging. Of course, there has been interest in aging processes by philosophers and natural scientist for far longer, at least since classical Greece and Rome (for example, Seneca's *De Senectutis*). In the 1700's, 1800's and early 1900's, some relatively scientific studies of aging were conducted, for example, by Quetelet, who was interested in mortality trends and in the "laws" of aging. In 1910 the psychologist G. Stanley Hall published *Senescence*, the first attempt to gather together knowledge about the aging process.

However, only at the end of World War Two did groups of researchers and practitioners gather together to discuss age and aging and to begin publications devoted specifically to gerontology. The Gerontological Society (of America), American Geriatrics Society, and International Association of Gerontology all began in the 1940's. Interestingly, the Gerontological Society was begun primarily by biologists and those in clinical medicine to be a research adjunct to geriatric applications: the focus was to do research on ways to "cure" aging. As years went by, though, the organization became more social in nature, mostly because of a need to investigate the effects of Social Security, retirement, housing, and social services. These research activities, in turn, were made urgent by the development of two sets of governmental programs: 1) those set up, especially in the Older Americans Act of 1965, to provide social service programs directly to older persons and 2) housing programs to build and support age-segregated public and non-profit housing for middle and lower income elderly (and disabled adults of all ages). Importantly for the history of gerontology, it was often based in a "social problems" orientation-- that is, it began with the assumption that older persons had unique, special problems that required unique, age-specific solutions.

Research and programs in aging from the 1960's through the 1970's expanded greatly as the elderly population increased. Research of all kinds, especially biomedical, was particularly defined and supported by the establishment of the National Institute on Aging in 1975. As with many governmental programs, social services, elderly housing, and research (to a much lesser degree) saw a dramatic downturn in the 1980's. In the 1990's NIA is recording relatively large increases in funding for research, mostly focused on health issues in later life but also including social research. Meanwhile, the composition of the Gerontological Society has shifted once again, this time toward psychology of aging, on the one hand, and practice on the other.

A SAMPLER OF ISSUES IN GERONTOLOGY

Cursory glimpses at just a few of the current areas of gerontological research will make the preceding discussions of concepts, methods, and history more concrete. A part of the rationale for selection is to represent major areas of current concern not represented in the annotated bibliographies. In this brief journey we will proceed from the small to the very large. We will begin with biological theories of aging and then touch upon physiological and sensory changes, perception, cognition, and personality at the individual level, also including consideration of the interplay between the individual and his or her physical environment. At the more macro-level of social gerontology, we will consider retirement and several aspects of the economics of aging. Those discussions, especially, will also touch upon a number of policy issues related to aging.

1. Theories of Biological Aging

Physiologists and biologists of aging, not surprisingly, have been interested in understanding the basic mechanisms underlying biological aging processes. Theories that are being tested for their contribution range from the smallest micro-level of analysis to explanations that are environmental in nature. Much of the investigation is on animal aging or laboratory analysis of tissues. For example, there is increasing evidence of a role for genetic programming in determining the maximum lifespan of the species (which appears to be about 140 years for humans) and the potential lifespan of an individual. There may be a genetic code that limits the number of times a cell replicates; once this is exceeded, the cell no longer reproduces. As more and more cells follow this path, larger and larger systems of the body can no longer function. A very different approach, the wear and tear theory, hypothesizes that environmental stressors inevitably take their toll over time. Even without a "built in" mechanism for death, the accumulation of insults to the body produces such a level of damage that the systems can no longer function adequately. From this theoretical vantage point, there is a direct relationship between the reduction of environmental stressors (from pollution to temperature extremes) and longer lifespans.

There are a range of theories between the micro-level of DNA and the relative macro-level of environmental insults (see, for example, Hayflick, 1987, for a review). The reality, certainly, is that aging and eventual death result from a broad set of interacting factors. Some of these factors are intrinsic to the organism, that is, are part of being a biological entity, whereas others are extrinsic to the individual organism. Many biologists and geriatricians find it convenient to try to separate the former factor-- called *primary aging*--from both environmental factors and the impact of particular disease states, labelled *secondary aging* (although others refer to aging as a disease process). Even when diseases are closely related to old age they are secondary if they are not an inevitable part of growing old.

2. Sensory and Perceptual Changes with Age

Another set of researchers in the areas of physiology and psychology study the ways that one's ability to sense and interact with the physical world change over time. It is clear that virtually all older persons experience a lessening of the effectiveness of their senses. Although this is not an appropriate place to go into the explanations of age changes in sensation and perception, suffice it to say that both primary and secondary aging seem to be involved and that both the peripheral systems (the outer organ systems) and central ones (the central nervous system-- CNS) are adversely affected.

Descriptively there are three major changes in virtually all bodily systems and functions that conspire to reduce not only sensation and perception but also movement and performance. These three can be roughly classified as: loss of speed, or slowing; loss of sharpness and acuity, or dulling; and loss of flexibility, or hardening. All three can have serious impact on activities and performance of older persons and all show up clearly on laboratory tests of performance, although it is important to realize that for most older persons they are not so severe that they have much day to day impact.

Loss of speed occurs throughout the aging body. In fact, one of the major explanations for biological aging emphasizes the fact that the central nervous system (CNS) slows down. Conduction of information from nerves to the brain, processing within the brain, and transmission of instructions from the brain to the sense organs all take longer in an older individual. There are many other losses of speed as well, for example, in the speed of adaptation of eyes and ears to changes in frequency and intensity of stimuli and in slowing in contraction of muscles and corresponding gross motor movement.

A loss of flexibility is also apparent in one's sensory systems with age. For example, the lenses of the eye harden, making it much more difficult to focus as well as producing glare in bright lights. The skin loses its flexibility, producing both a loss in sensitivity of touch and the flaccidity so often expressed in wrinkles, folds of loose skin under the arms, and even enlarged ears, especially in men.

Loss of acuity, likewise, is apparent in studies of all senses. In the CNS this loss of acuity is often expressed as a change in the signal to noise ratio for detecting information. Whenever anyone attempts to see, hear, or feel something, he or she must be able to screen out irrelevant or competing information coming from the senses so that perception can be concentrated on the signal, the desired, meaningful information. All of us sometimes have problems in this regard-- seeing an approaching car when there is movement behind it or the sun overhead, hearing what someone is saying while another person is making noise or an air conditioner is running nearby, and so on. Older persons have more difficulty picking the signal out from the noise, apparently for two reasons. On the one hand, they may be experiencing a greater amount of internal noise interfering with good perception, in that brain synapses may be firing on a random basis or input from two sources may be confused. On the other hand, they have less ability to differentiate two closely presented stimuli than younger persons do. An extensive series of studies on masking (presenting a second stimulus right before or after the signal to be attended to and seeing how that interferes with perception or comprehension of the signal) illustrate clearly the significant age differences in these areas.

Before leaving this topic, three important points should be made. First, almost all the research done on these topics is cross-sectional. Although there may be better reason in this area of research than in many others to believe that cohort and period effects are relatively minimal, caution still must be exercised. Second, even though results of comparing young to old are often statistically quite dramatic, they are still relatively small in relation both to the percentage of loss compared to intact ability and the likelihood that in most everyday situations neither the older nor the younger person needs to perform at the absolute limit of their ability (which is what is tested in the laboratory). As a result, often these differences make little difference in most regular activities. Third, many of the effects can be minimized by either prosthetics, such as hearing aids and glasses, or by changes in the environmental conditions so that situations that are particularly problematic are avoided or altered to eliminate their worst aspects, as in minimizing glare while still providing good lighting or sound-proofing a room.

3. Person/Environment Fit

The mention of changing environmental conditions leads to a third area of research in gerontology, that concerned with how older persons deal with their physical environments. It should come as no surprise that more older than younger persons have difficulty manipulating and using their physical settings. Any aspects of the physical environment that feed into the sensory deficits just considered will adversely affect elderly even if they do not present problems to younger persons. I sometimes refer to this as a "snowstorm effect," that is, older persons must regularly contend with a given environment in the ways younger persons might do in a snowstorm. They move more slowly, have to use greater effort to insure they are not doing something wrong or dangerous, and try to stay as "close to home" as possible (proximity effect).

Because of the importance of environmental characteristics to the everyday lives of older persons, many gerontologists have been interested in how older people relate to the physical environment. One of the most popular of several models is the ecological model of Lawton and Nahemow (1973). They state that both environments and persons can be placed on dimensions. Persons can range from having high to low ability to deal with various environmental demands; environments can be arrayed on a dimension from high to low demand. In other words, some environments demand a great deal of those who use them-- they must be strong, have very sharp senses, be agile, etc.-- while others demand much less. Likewise, some persons have a great amount of capability in those areas while others do not (although they may be comparable in many other ways). What is important is to have a relatively good match or fit between environmental demands and personal abilities. If the environment is too demanding, the person will be unable to cope adequately; if it is too simple and undemanding, it will be boring. One of the problems of aging is that people's abilities can change quite dramatically or decline slowly over time; in either case, an environment that was once fitting may become problematic. By the same token, placing the person in very undemanding environment, like a nursing home, as soon as they show any loss of capability, is likely to engender passivity and atrophy of skills.

These notions have been applied to housing environments and architectural design, as well as providing a paradigm for basic research on both personal characteristics and environmental elements. Thus, it is a good example of the importance of bringing together the basic and applied aspects of gerontology to mutual advantage.

4. Cognition and Intelligence

Perhaps the largest single area of research in gerontology in the last decade is that of the cognitive psychology of aging. Thousands of studies have examined how older persons process information, remember, learn, make decisions, and perform on intellectual tests. Several recent textbooks and monographs provide detailed coverage of these issues. In this space we will briefly consider, not the specifics of this research, but several research issues raised in this area.

As with other areas, much of the work on cognition and aging is cross-sectional; thus, the same issues already raised emerge once again. It has become clear that only some areas or aspects of cognitive processing appear to be of a primary aging nature. It is also known that training, getting people acclimated to the research experience, and a number of other "contextual" factors mitigate older-younger differences. The latter findings indicate that cohort factors related to recent experience with research, use of certain strategies, and flexibility in moving from one strategy to another are important elements in producing age group differences. Thus, the challenge for researchers is to separate the age/maturational effects from the cohort ones to be able to specify mechanisms that are intrinsically changing as people get older.

In fact, in few areas of gerontology is the importance of paying attention to cohort factors more obvious than in studies of intelligence. Intelligence, as defined in the research, is a relatively global concept in comparison to many of the specific mechanisms that are the focus of much cognitive research. Intelligence-- that is, performance on intelligence tests-- is a composite of many factors, ranging from basic perception to higher order reasoning to accessing a base of knowledge built up over years of experience. Early research on intelligence, in which older age groups performed much worse than younger ones in cross-sectional studies, led gerontologists to posit involved explanations of how and why age changes occur. However, when more careful sampling was done (including making sure to screen for disease-related intellectual losses that are differentially distributed across the age groups) and, especially, when longitudinal data were collected, something dramatic became clear: much of the so-called aging effect is really a cohort effect. Data from a number of sources, especially a longitudinal study by K. Warner Schaie and his colleagues (for example, Schaie, 1983) that is now almost a quarter of a century old, show that until quite late in life (70s and 80s), most persons perform about as well overall on intelligence tests as they did several decades earlier. The "deterioration" in earlier studies was, in fact, great differences in educational level, experience with test situations, and other factors that are not maturational or developmental.

Another aspect of intelligence testing has also become clear as more research has been done, and that is that there are several very distinct aspects of performance that become combined in calculation of overall intelligence scores. Different subscales of the tests differentially are linked to these facets of intelligence. A distinction that has been carefully explored is that between fluid and crystallized intelligence. Fluid intelligence is a process variable-- how people choose and apply various logical reasoning strategies to solve particular problems; crystallized intelligence is more the content of intelligence-- that which is known. Most studies comparing old and young have found that fluid intelligence measures show considerably greater age declines (even longitudinally) than do measures of crystallized intelligence, which in some cases show continued progress.

Intelligence studies, thus, clearly show both the importance of ruling out cohort factors when attempting to develop age explanations (or of directly examining how cohort expresses itself in performance) and the value of making appropriately fine distinctions in the measurement of dependent variables so that all appropriate dimensions can be examined. More generally, cognitive psychology is a fertile field for exploring the interplay of age, cohort, and period factors and for delineating the "mental performance" outcomes of the physiological changes already described.

5. Personality: Stable or Changing?

Another group of psychologists of aging focus on personality in later life. They are interested in defining the variation over time in people's characteristic ways of approaching situations and thinking about themselves and other people. As briefly noted early in this chapter, the area of personality is clearly divided into two major camps, one of which stresses continuity of personality and the other change over time. The latter group often specifies a set of personality factors that are posited to be specific to later life.

McCrae and Costa (1990) are the most well-known proponents of the continuity idea of personality. They have done considerable research using factor analytic and related techniques to show that there at least three major traits of personality: optimism/pessimism, introversion/extroversion, and neuroticism that are relatively stable from middle age to late adulthood.

On the other hand, many personality theorists are stage theorists; they maintain that as people move through life they take up different tasks that require them to act and think in qualitatively different ways. Theorists like Erikson, Levinson, Vaillant, Havighurst, and Gutmann, among others, characterize development precisely as movement through the stages (see McRae and Costa, 1990, and Wrightsman, 1986, for overviews). Several of these have described later life as a period of greater introspection (sometimes labeled "interiority" and passivity). Gutmann (1987, in particular, states that men become more intimacy-oriented and women more achievement-oriented as they age.

These two positions appear to be contradictory. Much of the contradiction is more apparent than real, and much of it derives from different research goals and different methods to achieve those goals. In fact, everyone agrees that there is both change and stability of variables encompassed by "personality" as people move through life; stability or change are a matter of emphasis, not exclusivity. McCrae and Costa rely almost exclusively on personality scales-- closed ended measures as described earlier-- which measure very global "orientations to the world." It is unlikely that such measures would tap into the phenomenological dynamics of self-definition or the ways people respond differently to specific situations as they age. Most of the stage theorists (and others, such as dialectical theorists--see Riegel, 1976), on the other hand, use case studies and extensive interview procedures to develop qualitative "portraits" of aging. These methods are more sensitive to changing definitions of self than the more global methodologies of personality scale advocates. Aging is likely to present a changing array of opportunities and experiences that are likely to result in change over time, but it is also built upon the foundation of the earlier parts of life and, thus, allows individuals to make use of the characteristic action patterns they have developed through their previous interactions with others and times of self-contemplation.

6. Retirement

Retirement research forms a transition between more micro-level studies such as the previous examples and macro-level analyses. On both levels, it is illustrative of the influence of cohort and period effects.

Even though the lifespan has been increasing, the age at retirement has been declining. This trend amplifies the effects of the considerably larger percentage of the population that is above the age of 60. Currently, the average age at retirement is merely 61 years, meaning that many people will spend almost as many years after retirement as they did in the work force. Macro-level gerontologists have been studying the impact of this phenomenon on society. Some policy analysts and politicians have pointed to dire effects on the economy, while others have indicated that other competing trends, such as fewer children, and the ability of many retirees to be active, contributing members of society make such negative predictions unlikely. In any case, sociologists, economists, and political scientists of aging have directed major research efforts toward documenting the current state of affairs and predicting the contours and the effects as large future cohorts retire.

Macro-level work is complemented by studies on the effects of retiring on individuals. Early research on the personal effects of retirement in the 1950's and 1960's indicated a number of negative outcomes. In fact, some research intimated that retirement caused illness and death because people who retired were found to die at younger ages than those who continued to work. More recent research (for example, Parnes et al, 1985; Williamson, Rinehart, and Blank, 1992), on the other hand, is virtually unanimous in showing that the vast majority of retirees (approximately 85%) are as happy or happier being retired than they were when working. Also, whereas some of the explanations given for the earlier negative effects stressed that those resulted from lack of continued activity--thus, leading to predictions that finding other work or involvement in volunteer activities would soften the blow of retirement-- most recent research indicates little or no effect of returning to work or volunteering on satisfaction with retirement.

How can these findings be reconciled? Much clearly has to do with period effects. In the 1950's and 1960's people usually retired for one of two reasons: because retirement at a certain age was mandated or because they were too ill to continue to work. Obviously, if one is too ill to work he or she is going to be quite unhappy; also, he or she is likely to die earlier than someone who is of comparable age but healthy, providing an explanation for the supposed link between retirement and premature death.

At this time, most people retire because they feel they have worked long enough (or, in these recessionary times, because their employer offered an inducement to leave the work force). The most important predictor of retirement satisfaction is a belief that one will have sufficient income to live about as comfortably in retirement as one had while working. These reasons to retire are not likely to make people negative about the event of retiring. At the same time, retirement has moved from a relatively new transition, seen as signalling the "end of the line," to an expectable event, often interpreted as being the entry into a new phase of leisure. These period effects result in a more positive overall evaluation of retirement on the part of individuals, and when those individuals are aggregated lead to a general positive social view of retirement.

7. Economics of Aging

Another area of macro-societal research on aging is related to the retirement studies just cited, but is focused on the question of the economic status of the aged. Again, research findings and policy applications are co-mingled, as bureaucrats decide whether or not to institute or cut back on income support policies to the elderly.

Most studies of the economics of aging indicate a success story for American governmental programs. As recently as thirty years ago, the percentage of elderly that was below the poverty line was much higher than that of the population in general. In response to that terrible situation, federally instituted programs were enacted, ranging from enhancements to Social Security and Medicare to Supplemental Security Income to provision of services directly to elders through the Area Agencies on Aging network. Combined with better pension programs and other factors, these initiatives resulted in a slightly lower level of poverty in elderly than in the population as a whole (and a significantly lower one than families with small children). This state of affairs has spawned calls for "generational equity," which essentially means cutting back on programs for the elderly and using those resources for programs for children.

Economists of aging (Schulz, 1985) and analysts of aging policy (Wisensale, 1988), however, have argued that the statistics about elderly and poverty are somewhat misleading. If a somewhat higher target is used, such as 150% of the poverty level, elderly are more likely than other groups to fall into the low income category. Further, part of the reason for the relatively good economic situation of the elderly is the presence of the very income maintenance programs, such as Supplemental Security Income, that are targeted by the generational equity proponents. Again, we can see how data can be interpreted in several ways depending upon one's basic assumptions and goals and how research results interplay with practice, in this case policy determinations.

ACCESS: GERONTOLOGY

This chapter has provided a review of basic concepts, methods, and issues in gerontology and furnished brief glimpses into research findings that span the "road map" of disciplinary interests that compose gerontology. Subsequent chapters will provide considerable detail about selected topics. While this chapter merely scratches the surface of gerontology, the bibliographic chapters that follow do not flesh out every part of this skeleton, for no single book can begin to cover all aspects of an area as varied as gerontology.

Before proceeding to a description of the approach used in the remainder of the book, let us consider a few places to look for more detailed discussions of gerontology as a whole, including textbooks, handbooks and related reference documents, and journals. The sources mentioned are just a few of the most well-known and accessible in the field that is growing by the month; almost every major textbook publisher has at least one gerontology text in its current list, and new handbooks and scholarly monographs are constantly appearing.

Texts

The 1980's saw a proliferation of good basic introductory texts in gerontology, a trend that has continued in the 1990's with revisions of the "standards" as well as new entries. The basic texts can be roughly divided into two categories: some of the texts are more oriented toward "social gerontology," comprising the more macro-level end of the field, whereas others place more emphasis on the biological and psychological micro-level. All of those listed, however, give at least some background to most of the major areas of gerontology. Some of the more widely used are:

More "social gerontological":

Atchley, Robert C., Social Forces and Aging (6 ed.), Wadsworth,
    1991;
Hooyman, Nancy, and Kiyak, H. Asuman, Social Gerontology: A
    Multidisciplinary Perspective (2 ed.), Allyn and Bacon,
    1988;

More psychological/biological:

Botwinick, Jack, Aging and Behavior (3 ed.), 1984, Springer;
Cavanaugh, John C., Adult Development and Aging (2 ed.), 1993,
    Brooks/Cole;
Kimmel, Douglas C., Adulthood and Aging (3 ed.), 1990, Wiley;
Schaie, K. Warner, and Willis, Sherry L., Adult Development and
    Aging (3 ed.), 1991, HarperCollins;
Stevens-Long, Judith, and Commons, Michael, Adulthood and Aging (4
    ed.), 1992, Mayfield.

Handbooks, Encyclopedias, and Other Reference Sources

The most comprehensive and most widely-cited handbooks are the three volume sets of Handbooks put out by Van Nostrand Reinhold, now in their third editions. They are directed primarily to graduate student and professional audiences. Each edition includes: Handbook of Biology of Aging, Handbook of Psychology of Aging, and Handbook of Aging and the Social Sciences. The first editions came out in the mid-1970's, the second in 1985, and the most recent in 1990. The third editions are edited by Edward L. Schneider and John W. Rowe, James E. Birren and K. Warner Schaie, and Robert H. Binstock and Linda K. George, respectively. I would recommend using the second edition in conjunction with the third. Some areas covered in the second edition do not appear in the third, while some chapters in the third edition are quite abbreviated to update the area between 1985 and 1990 rather than to provide a comprehensive review on their own.

Another major handbook is the Handbook of Clinical Gerontology, edited by Carstensen and Edelstein in 1987. It provides relatively brief overviews in five major sections, covering normal aging, psychiatric disorders, behavioral problems, and social issues. Also a good reference source is the Annual Review of Gerontology and Geriatrics series. Now in its eleventh volume, this yearly compendium provides detailed coverage of specialized areas. Although any given year does not give as full an overview as the handbooks, taken together the set includes major reviews of most areas within gerontology (and, obviously, geriatrics). For example, volume 10 is entirely concerned with biological aspects of aging.

Two recent encyclopedias are relevant to gerontologists as well. Both give succinct definitions of major concepts and summaries of knowledge about a wide range of topics. The Encyclopedia of Aging, edited by George L. Maddox and others (1987), is particularly comprehensive. The Encyclopedia of Adult Development, edited by Robert Kastenbaum (forthcoming), includes consideration of aging issues, although it is explicitly focused on adult development as a lifespan process and, so, ties gerontology into broader adult issues.

Major Journals

A count made by Johanne Philbrick for her dissertation (1991) revealed 112 journals with primarily gerontological content published in the United States alone. Many of these are highly specialized journals with small circulations. Several major journals in the field are briefly described below.

The Gerontologist is an official publication of the Gerontological Society of America. It is directed toward the society membership as a whole. The primary focus is on practice and organizational issues, but it also regularly includes research reports as long as they have direct practical significance.

The Journal of Gerontology is the other major Gerontological Society publication and the most-cited research journal in gerontology. It is divided into four sections: Biological Sciences, Clinical Medicine, Psychological Sciences, and Social Sciences. Virtually all of the studies reported are experimental in nature, and many are quite specialized.

Psychology and Aging is published by the American Psychological Association. Now in its sixth year, it is a major outlet for psychological research articles. Research on Aging, on the other hand, is more sociologically-oriented, while Experimental Aging Research is more biological and very experimental in focus. Journal of Aging Studies is a recently-begun outlet for articles that are more qualitative or utilize unusual methods. The International Journal of Aging and Human Development presents a wider variety of articles in the behavioral and social sciences of aging than either of those journals. Journal of Applied Gerontology also ranges quite widely in disciplinary orientation but publishes articles with direct application to gerontological practice. Aging is published by the federal Administration on Aging and features short presentations of recent findings. Of course, non-gerontological journals in sociology, psychology, economics, medicine, and many other areas occasionally include articles about aging.

Information about articles in both large and small gerontological journals and many of those that are not specifically gerontological is included in the

Ageline database available in many university and public libraries. It is particularly strong in the areas of psychological and social gerontology, but less useful for biological science interests. For those interested in the more social and behavioral science end of gerontology, an excellent way to find one's way through the journals is to do a keyword search using Ageline.

CONCLUSION

Gerontology, then, is a widely ranging field of study, encompassing almost every point in the constellation of academic disciplines. Gerontologists may work in experimental laboratories or other cultures, using highly advanced technological devices or nothing but a pad and pencil and a set of ideas. They may confine themselves to basic science research or extend themselves to a wide variety of practical applications of their own research and that of their peers. They may identify closely with a "home discipline" or see themselves as carving out a new and different, interdisciplinary field.

In spite of all this variety, they have a great amount in common. They are all focused upon the two major ways of considering aging discussed at the beginning of this chapter-- the state of being old and the process of aging. They are all faced with trying to account not only for age and change in individuals but also for the changing contexts of aging-- placement in space and movement in time. They are part of an exciting, challenging, and changing profession, one that is itself far from elderly. The fruits of their work are just beginning to be seen in many areas of academia and everyday life.

Because of the diversity of gerontology, it is important for all who are part of the enterprise-- researchers, theorists, educators, practitioners, and students alike-- to be guided by an appreciation of their diversity and their common goals, to see the forest and the trees. The terrain of gerontology is broad and deep and the trails can sometimes be winding (and not well marked); the road map of the disciplines and the topics can be a guide for placing the much more specific considerations of any one group of gerontologists into perspective.

REFERENCES

Association for Gerontology in Higher Education. (1991). National Directory of Educational Programs in Gerontology. Washington, D. C.: Association for Gerontology in Higher Education.
Baltes, P. B., Reese, H. W., & Nesselroade, J. R. (1977). Life-span Developmental Psychology: Introduction to Research Methods. Monterey, CA: Brooks-Cole.

Carstensen, L. L., & Edelstein, B. A. (1987). Handbook of Clinical Gerontology. New York: Pergamon.

Elder, G. H. (1974). Children of the Great Depression: Social Change and Life Experiences. Chicago: University of Chicago Press.

Gutmann, D. L. (1987). Reclaimed Powers: Toward a New Psychology of Men and Women in Later Life. New York: Basic.

Hayflick, L. (1987). Biological theories of aging. In G. L. Maddox (Ed.), The Encyclopedia of Aging. New York: Springer.

Kastenbaum, R. J. (forthcoming). The Encyclopedia of Adult Development. Phoenix, AZ: Oryx.

Lawton, M. P., & Nahemow, L. (1973). Ecology and the aging process. In C. Eisdorfer & M. P. Lawton (Eds.), The Psychology of Adult Development and Aging (pp. 619-674). Washington: American Psychological Association.

Maddox, G. L. (1987). The Encyclopedia of Aging. New York: Springer.

McRae, R. R., & Costa, P. T. (1990). Personality in Adulthood. New York: Guilford.

Parnes, H. S., Crowley, J. E., Haurin, R. J., Less, L. J., Morgan, W. R., Mott, F. L., & Nestel, G. (1985). Retirement among American Men. Lexington, MA: Lexington.

Philbrick, J. (1991). Journals in Gerontology: The Art of a Science. Unpublished doctoral dissertation, University of Connecticut.

Riegel, K. F. (1976). The dialectics of human development. American Psychologist, 31, 689-700.

Schaie, K. W. (1965). A general model for the study of developmental problems. Psychological Bulletin, 64, 92-107.

Schaie, K. W. (1983). Longitudinal Studies of Adult Psychological Development. New York: Guilford.

Schulz, J. H. (1985). The Economics of Aging (2 ed.). Belmont, CA: Wadsworth.

Williamson, R. C., Rinehart, A. N., & Blank, T. O. (1992). Early Retirement: Promises and Pitfalls. New York: Insight.

Wisensale, S. K. (1988). Generational equity and intergenerational policies. The Gerontologist, 28, 773-778.

Wrightsman, L. S. (1986). Personality development in adulthood. Monterey, CA: Brooks-Cole.

TOPICS
IN
GERONTOLOGY

1

HISTORY OF GERONTOLOGY

Johanne Philbrick

INTRODUCTION

As a science develops and matures, it begins to take more interest in its history and in a record of its evolution and growth. A solid base of knowledge built upon the past is a fundamental requisite of orderly growth. An historical record provides a science with an understanding of past development and a sense of future direction.

In order to have a clear understanding of the history of gerontology, it is necessary to consider the broader issue of the history of aging. An integrated approach to gerontological history must examine and weigh societal influences that created the need for a new science of aging. Historical gerontology is complex as it must reach backward to retrieve its rudiments from many academic disciplines: biology, medicine, sociology, psychology, and social work. Each of these disciplines has played a role in the development of the study of aging. To prevent the likelihood that these areas of interest might each grow in singular and disparate directions, a means was needed that would form a bond among the different disciplines and attempt to create order and continuity. This role in history was filled by the establishment of the Gerontological Society of America and its clinical contemporary, the American Geriatrics Society. The history of gerontology is intrinsically interwoven with the formation and advancement of these Societies. Their activities and publications are the major vehicle through which an interdisciplinary science of aging developed. These two interactive forces, the need for an interdisciplinary study of aging and a means by which to attain it, generated research and critical literature that defined the "state of the art" in gerontology today.

This bibliography identifies these three general areas of the history of gerontology: the need, the means, and the result. An annotated bibliography intended to help the reader explore the growth and expansion of gerontology must consider the contribution of each of these influences. The need is investigated through works that describe the broad, general experience of growing old in the United States and the beginnings of aging as a field of study. The means is traced through the history and development of the Gerontological Society of America and the American Geriatrics Society. The result is examined by exploring the historical research, criticism, and literature generated by the formation of a new science of aging. Citations relevant to more than one area are classified in the category of their main focus and notation is made of multiple emphasis.

RELATED READINGS

The Need

Butler, R. N. (1975). Why survive? Being old in America. New York: Harper & Row.

Calhoun, R. B. (1978). In search of the new old: Redefining old age in America, 1945-1970. New York: Elsevier.

Cowgill, D., & Holmes, L. (1972). Aging and modernization. New York: Appleton-Century-Crofts.

Cumming, E., & Henry, W. E. (1961). Growing old. New York: Basic.

Freeman, J. T. (1979). Aging. Its history and literature. New York: Human Sciences Press.

Freeman, J. T. (1965). Medical perspectives in aging (12th-19th century). The Gerontologist, 5, 1-24.

Hunter, A. (1980). Why Chicago? American Behavioral Scientist, 24, 215-227.

Kuhn, T. S. (1970). The structure of scientific revolutions (2nd ed.). Chicago: University of Chicago Press.

Shock, N. W. (1957). Trends in gerontology (2nd ed.). Stanford, CA: Stanford University Press.

The Means

Cole, T. R. (1984). The prophecy of senescence: G. Stanley Hall and the reconstruction of old age in America. The Gerontologist, 24, 360-366.

Cowdry, E. V. (1953). The Gerontological Society, its present and future. Journal of Gerontology, 8, 498-502.

Hedback, A. E. (1946). Good old age. Geriatrics, 1, 87-88.

Hinman, F. (1946). The dawn of gerontology. Journal of Gerontology, 1, 412-419.

Postell, W. D. (1946). Some American contributions to the literature of geriatrics. Geriatrics, 1, 41-45.

Riegel, K. (1977). A history of psychological gerontology. In J. E. Birren & K. W. Schaie (Eds.), Handbook of the psychology of aging (pp. 70-102). New York: Van Nostrand Reinhold.

Thompson, W. O. (1953). Aging comes of age. Journal of the American Geriatrics Society, 1, 1-2.

Tuohy, E. L. (1946). Geriatrics: The general setting. Geriatrics, 1, 17-20.

The Result

Abrahams, J. P., Hoyer, W. J., Elias, M. F., Bradigan, B. (1975). Gerontological research in psychology published in the Journal of Gerontology 1963-1974: Perspectives and progress. Journal of Gerontology, 30, 668-673.

Achenbaum, W. A. (1987). Can gerontology be a science? Journal of Aging Studies, 1, 3-18.

Birren, J. E. (1968). Research on aging: A frontier of science and social gain. The Gerontologist, 8, 7-13.

Birren, J. E. (1962). Fifteen annual meetings later. The Gerontologist, 2, 179-181.

Birren, J. E., & Cunningham, W. R. (1985). Research on the psychology of aging. In J. E. Birren & K. W. Schaie (Eds.), Handbook of the psychology of aging (2nd ed.) (pp. 3-38). New York: Van Nostrand Reinhold.

Cole, T. R. (1988). Aging, history, and health: Progress and paradox. In J. J. F. Schroots, J. E. Birren & A. Svanborg (Eds.), Health and aging: Perspectives and Prospects (pp. 45-63). New York: Springer.

Estes, C. (1980). The aging enterprise. San Francisco: Jossey-Bass.

Gitman, L. (1963). Is the Gerontological Society necessary? The Gerontologist, 3, 98-99.

Kastenbaum, R. (1978). Essay: Gerontology's search for understanding. The Gerontologist, 18, 59-63.

Kleemeier, R. W. (1965). Gerontology as a discipline. The Gerontologist, 5, 237-239, 276.

Morris, R. (1967). The Gerontological Society's contribution to public policy - Reality or illusion. The Gerontologist, 7, 229-233.

Poon, L. W., & Welford, A. T. (1980). Prologue. A historical perspective. In L. W. Poon (Ed.), Aging in the 1980s (pp. xiii-xvii). Washington, DC: American Psychological Association.

Pratt, H. J. (1976). The gray lobby. Chicago: University of Chicago Press.

Riegel, K. (1977). Past and future trends in gerontology. The Gerontologist, 17, 105-113.

Seltzer, M. M. (1983). Unstarted projects, unused paragraphs, and unfinished business. The Gerontologist, 23, 120-22.

Shock, N. W. (1951). A classified bibliography of gerontology and geriatrics. Stanford: Stanford University Press.

Van Tassel, D. D. (1978). Symposium: Role of humanities in gerontology. The Gerontologist, 18, 574-583 (with S. J. Kleinberg, M. Sohngen, S. F. Spicker, W. G. Moss).

ANNOTATED BIBLIOGRAPHY

The Need

1-1. Achenbaum, W. A. (1978). Old age in the new land: The American experience since 1790. Baltimore, MD: John Hopkins.

Achenbaum's book provides a valuable, insightful examination of the history of old age in America. It analyzes the changing status of the elderly in the course of the nation's history. The underlying theme of the text is an inversion of values in American society. Achenbaum believes that constancy and change in attitudes toward the elderly have been the result of both inherent beliefs about the assets and liabilities of old age and prevailing conditions and values in American culture from 1790 to the present. From the Civil War to World War I, the changing position of the elderly is traced as an historical era in which older people's worth was increasingly devalued in conjunction with a heightened response to the value and importance of youth. Assets previously ascribed to the old gradually came to be associated with the young. Wisdom became intelligence; power became strength; and experience was replaced by being attuned to "modern conditions." After World War I, a tough realism hell-bent on progress undermined the traditional functions of older people. Guardians of the past became obsolescent in a society increasingly oriented toward the future. The book successfully exposes the falseness of the stereotypes attributed to older people as the society became increasingly aligned with the potential of youth.

1-2. Birren, J. E. (1961). A brief history of the psychology of aging. The Gerontologist, 1, Part I 69-77, Part II 127-134.

These two papers cover a time span of 125 years beginning in 1835 and ending in 1960. These years are divided into three distinct historical periods: the Early Period from 1835 to 1918, Beginning Systematic Studies from 1918 to 1940, and The Period of Expansion from 1946 to 1960. There is a gap between 1940 and 1946 as all study and research was put on hold when the entire intent and thrust of the nation was dedicated to the World War II effort. In the Early Period, Quetelet, who was born in Ghent in 1796, was the first to begin to gather statistics on the regularities of aging and analyze this collected data mathematically. It is he who developed the concept of the average man around which other values and measurements could be distributed. Quetelet's work attracted and influenced Galton, an English geographer who evolved into an anthropologist and later a psychologist. Galton's anthropometric studies,

Inquiries into Human Faculty and Its Development (1883), was the first definitive work in developmental psychology. The period from 1918 to 1940, classified as Beginning Systematic Studies, begins with the work of G. Stanley Hall (1844-1924). Hall's book, *Senescence, the Last Half of Life*, published in 1922, tried to find meaning and value in the later years of life. In this book, Hall reached into the future to call out for a scientific study of aging at a time when psychologists were interested almost exclusively in childhood. By the mid 1930's, psychologists had begun to see aging as a time of life worthy of comprehensive study and analytical experiments. By 1940, the study of psychological aging had become systematic and institutionalized. The Period of Expansion from 1946 to 1960 saw the rapid development of research laboratories devoted to aging, the initiation of professional, scientific aging societies, national and international conferences, and, perhaps most important, a new breed of psychologist whose career and life work was centered in the processes of aging. A Gerontology Unit was established as part of the National Institutes of Health and an International Association of Gerontology was formed to coordinate research from around the world. Universities established Aging Centers and began to offer courses designed to train students in aging studies. Research publications in psychological aging grew from Quetelet's one and only in 1835 to more than 300 from 1950 to 1959. Through the years, the psychology of aging came of age expanding from one lone scholar in 1835 to a White House Conference on Aging in 1961. Birren's personal knowledge of many of the events and persons in the later years adds special insight to these papers.

1-3. Birren, J. E., & Clayton, V. (1975). History of gerontology. In J. E. Birren & D. S. Woodruff (Eds.), <u>Aging: Scientific perspectives and social issues</u> (pp. 15-17). New York: D. Van Nostrand.

This chapter presents a brief history of the development of gerontology as a science. The authors discuss three themes around which myths about aging developed and the ways in which present research can be related to these basic themes. The *antediluvian* theme arose from the belief that in earlier times people lived to reach phenomenal old ages. The book of Genesis records Adam's life span as 930 years, Seth as 912 years, and Noah as 950 years. Examples of such extended life also appear in the beliefs and folklore of other cultures. A second theme, the *hyperborean*, is based on the premise that in some distant, remote areas people live for a remarkably long time. A third theme, the *rejuvenation* theme, evolved around legends that somewhere there exists an elixir that will, if it can only be found, grant eternal youth. Each of these themes extols the prolongation of life. The authors believe that some aspects of past and current research are related to the pursuit of longevity and rejuvenation set forth in these age old beliefs about old age. Historical data touch upon the history of gerontology from the beginning of the scientific era in the 1600's through the tremendous growth in gerontological interest in the 1900's. The chapter is particularly valuable in the attention it gives to the people who were important in the development of attitudes toward the aged and in the founding of a new science of aging.

1-4. Fischer, D. H. (1978). Growing old in America. New York: Oxford University Press.

This book is an easily readable discussion of the "fall of the elderly from grace." Fischer begins with the premise that old age was an exalted position in early America. Fundamental changes in American culture and values from 1770 to 1970 led to a revolution in age relations and the development of a cult of youth in modern America. A combination of demographics and countervailing tendencies in American society created a situation in which old age was devalued to first a personal problem and then a social problem. Fischer's theme, based on the dubious premise that the elderly were revered in Colonial America, is that, as youth gained predominance, the aged were increasingly disesteemed and scorned. In turn, as the numbers of elderly grew significantly, older people came to be viewed as a social and political "problem." Fischer concludes that it was neither modernization, industrialization, nor urbanization that caused the forfeiture of high status for the elderly, but rather confrontation between the authority of one generation over another and the autonomy of individuals within them. Fundamental changes in world culture occurred in which authoritarian societies broke down and were supplanted by ideals of liberty and equality. The cult of old age was overthrown by an emerging ideal of age equality. What the book lacks in depth, it more than compensates for with its engaging literary style.

1-5. Frank, L. K. (1946). Gerontology. Journal of Gerontology, 1, 1-11.

This is the first article from the first publication of the Journal of Gerontology. It presents a comprehensive discussion of current issues in aging at that time. The growth of gerontology is traced as emerging in response to the misuse and neglect of older people. The article discusses gerontology as an academic discipline and as an applied science. It reflects on appropriate methods to meet the new problems posed by an aging population in a society altered by historical change. Biological and clinical aspects of aging are considered in conjunction with the social milieu. In this early writing, Frank makes a cogent argument supporting the need for provisions for care of the elderly, access to individual services, and the adoption of a national policy to direct the development of future social, economic, and political programs. The new Journal of Gerontology, as the first interdisciplinary regularly printed medium in the field, is rightly prophesied as a vehicle which will provide the needed means of communication to enable disparate disciplines to work together. This article and its companion introductory article, "Geriatrics" by E. J. Stieglitz (1946), should be read together.

1-6. Freeman, J. T. (1980). Historical note: Some notes on the history of the National Institute on Aging. The Gerontologist, 20, 610-614.

This article traces recognition of the need for a national organization devoted exclusively to issues and problems of aging. As early as 1896, individual efforts had attempted to further this goal. The author reviews the history of federal involvement in health from the establishment of a Marine Hospital Service for Merchant Seamen in 1798 during the presidency of John Adams through the signing of the law on May 31, 1974 of the Research Aging Act that created The National Institute on Aging as a part of the National Institutes of Health. Two special points of interest in the article are its discussion of concurrent developments that influenced the establishment of The National Institute and the inclusion of the recommendations of the Gerontological Society to the White House Conference on Aging in 1961. Briefly, these recommendations proposed: (1) federal support for graduate training in gerontology, (2) long-term support, as much as 10-20 years, for studies on aging, (3) the establishment of centers on aging in universities, hospitals, and research institutions, (4) the establishment of an Institute of Gerontology within the National Institutes of Health, (5) federal support for the construction of research laboratories, and (6) federal support to evaluate the effectiveness of specific programs. It is telling, in retrospect, to consider the implementation of these recommendations.

1-7. Haber, C. (1983). Beyond sixty-five: The dilemma of old age in America's past. New York: Cambridge University Press.

As people become well advanced in years, they eventually reach a point where they are forced to withdraw from society. Haber describes this stage of life and names the state of being too old "superannuated." The book is especially relevant in its discussion of the influence of the medical or disease model of growing old on attitudes toward the elderly and the stereotypes that developed from these attitudes. The medical profession, social workers and planners, and providers of formal support all tended to emphasize the limitations of the elderly rather than their capabilities. Haber believes that this emphasis on decrement created our current models of old age and is still a strong influence on the beliefs we hold today. Social and political thought in the late nineteenth and early twentieth century changed the regimen of policies and programs for people of all ages from a criterion of functional ability to a bureaucratic criterion of chronological age, which, in turn, compartmentalized and structured the life course of Americans from youth in classrooms to the elderly in forced retirement. The book is among the first to draw an analogy between medical treatment of the post-climacteric stage of life as a time of loss of vital energy, deterioration, and an increased tendency toward insanity, which in turn led to justification for separating the elderly from work through retirement and eventually from family through institutionalization. Many of the ideas in this book are novel and the author is adept at convincing the reader of their legitimacy.

1-8. Stieglitz, E. J. (1946). Geriatrics. Journal of Gerontology, 1, 153-163.

This article outlines the place of geriatrics in the science of medicine and the relationship of geriatrics to the broader science of gerontology. The article and its companion piece, L. K. Franks's "Gerontology," provide an excellent contrast between gerontology and geriatrics in philosophy and future goals that helps to explain the different development of the two disciplines. At this point in history, Stieglitz sees the science of gerontology divided into three components: the biology of senescence, geriatrics, and the social, economic, and cultural problems of older people. Interestingly, it would be many years later that practice concepts and direct service were included under this broad umbrella. Geriatrics is approached from both the viewpoints of prevention and maintenance. The nature of geriatric patients and medical problems and symptoms endemic to the aged are discussed with detail unusual in such a short piece. The author also reviews disorders in later life, the major limitations in geriatric knowledge at this point in time, and the future potential of the "infant" science of geriatrics. In conclusion, goals are set for the future of geriatrics in research and for the application of geriatric advances to prolonged health and usefulness in old age. (cf. L. K. Frank, "Gerontology.")

The Means

1-9. Achenbaum, W. A. (1987). Reconstructing GSA's history. The Gerontologist, 27, 21-29.

Achenbaum's article offers an historical synopsis of the first forty years of the Gerontological Society of America. The Society was founded in 1946 as an outgrowth of the Club for Research on Ageing, an early organization formed to abet the publication of E. V. Cowdry's *Problems of Ageing* (1939). The focus of the article is both historical and evaluative. The author reviews the goals set forth as necessary objectives to support the need for an aging society and examines the degree and extent to which these goals have been fulfilled. The article traces the history, activities, and goals of the Society and compares and contrasts the intellectual and organizational development of gerontology and the Gerontological Society with concurrent trends in other natural and social sciences. Achenbaum lists past presidents and discusses the direction and implication of papers accepted by the Society for publication across the forty year period. The role of the Gerontological Society in the public policy arena is examined as well as the Society's influence on aging policies at the Federal level. The author proposes astute and far-reaching questions that prompt examination of past and future policies for individual members and the Society as a whole. The article is a good example of the use of the past as a heuristic device in planning for the future and should be read as both an historical record of the "means" and a telling analysis of the "results."

1-10. Adler, M. (1958). History of Gerontological Society, Inc. Journal of Gerontology, 13, 94-102.

Marjorie Lawson Adler was Administrative Secretary of the Gerontological Society for thirty years. Her article records the history of the Society from personal knowledge. Its chronological discussion describes early beginnings, incorporation, the founding of the *Journal of Gerontology* and the *Newsletter*, and the role that individuals and supporting Foundations played in the growth of aging as a science. The article begins with the formation of the Club for Research on Ageing in the 1930's and proceeds to discuss the beginning of the Gerontological Society, the assistance of the Josiah Macy Jr. Foundation, and the *Journal of Gerontology* with its soon defunct Non-Technical Supplement. The author's knowledge of past events provides a wealth of detail that is indispensable in exploring the development, structure, and institutionalization of gerontology. Adler's work is a treasure chest of the past that captures the finest points of the early history of gerontology. In reading the article a generation after it was written, one finds a prosaic style seldom seen today -- an orderly listing of factual events. The value of Adler's work is demonstrated by its citation in almost every publication that has been written on the history of gerontology.

1-11. Blumenthal, H. T. (1965). The shape of the Gerontological Society. The Gerontologist, 5, 2-3, 48.

Blumenthal suggests that, in spite of claims to the contrary, the Gerontological Society is multidisciplinary rather than interdisciplinary.

Biologists, sociologists, psychologists, and physicians generally speak only to their like. The different sections of the Society seldom work together, and, when they do, communication tends to be awkward. The author believes that a gradual consolidation of the separate sections of the Society would lead toward a more integrated approach to gerontological knowledge. Interdisciplinary programming procedures, referring to such as symposia and annual meetings, are not enough. The structure of the Society must be consolidated and Sectional identities put aside in order to achieve interdisciplinary aims and fulfill the common goal of the Society. Although the article was written almost thirty years ago, it is especially interesting and relevant in respect to the recent move by the Gerontological Society to divide the *Journal of Gerontology* into four separate sections, each with its own disciplinary emphasis. Blumenthal provides a cogent argument for the alternative of an integrated approach.

1-12. Freeman, J. T. (1961). Gerontology and the Gerontological Society. The Gerontologist, 1, 162-167.

This article, published in the first issue of *The Gerontologist* in 1961, describes and discusses the status of gerontology at that historical point in time. Freeman reviews the White House Conference on Aging, funding, custodial homes, social welfare as a scientific category, and the relationship between economics and clinical medicine. Additional commentary discusses the sections of the Gerontological Society, its publications, documentation of the field by Nathan Shock, and international study and research. The article examines the scope and limitations of the *Journal of Gerontology* and the expansion of the *Newsletter* to a new journal, *The Gerontologist*, and questions whether this might be an evasive step taken to placate publication aspirations of non-scientific components of the Society. The author sees Sectional monasticism as self-defeating in its failure to fulfill the philosophy of the Society's founding fathers. Freeman emphasizes the need for unity among scientific disciplines and a correlation between developments in geriatrics and gerontology. The historical value of this article is enhanced by the opportunity it provides for a comparison of the state of gerontology in 1961 and similarities and differences thirty years later.

1-13. Freeman, J. T. (1984). Edmund Vincent Cowdry, Creative Gerontologist: Memoir and biographical notes. The Gerontologist, 24, 641-645.

The article discusses the life and work of the eminent gerontologist, Edmund Vincent Cowdry. In many respects, Cowdry's life was synonymous with the development of gerontology as a scientific field of study. The beginning of the idea for a Gerontological Society and the publication of the Society's first *Newsletter* are historically interwoven with Cowdry's life.

Cowdry was a pioneer in the study of aging. His efforts were instrumental in the founding of the "Club for Research on Ageing" which culminated in the publication of three editions of *Problems of Ageing*, the first major interdisciplinary text in the field. Included in the article is a short autobiography written by Cowdry at Freeman's request. The autobiography details the development of gerontology and the contributions of many people in the field from the 1930's through the 1960's. The first person format of this autobiographical record provides a personalized document, an "I was there and this was how it was" tone seldom found in more formal historical literature.

1-14. Thewlis, M. W. (1953). History of the American Geriatrics   Society. Journal of the American Geriatrics Society, 1, 3-8.

On June 11, 1942, a concerned group of biologists and clinicians, under the guidance of Malcolm W. Thewlis, met at the Hotel Brighton in Atlantic City and formalized their association by establishing the American Geriatrics Society. The objective of the Society was to study clinical geriatric problems, including causes, prevention, and treatment of diseases, the rehabilitation of older patients, and to disseminate the knowledge gained from study and research. In contrast to the Gerontological Society, in which full participation was open to all, the Geriatrics Society limited its voting rights to physicians. Doctors of Philosophy were eligible to join but had no votes. Thewlis reviews the minutes of the first nine annual meetings, discusses growth in membership through the years, and offers some details on the beginning of the publication of the Society's own journal, the *Journal of the American Geriatrics Society*. The article is scant on relevant information. Unfortunately, the American Geriatrics Society, unlike the Gerontological Society, did not have an administrative secretary with the prudence to record the finer details of its early history. Short selections written by W. O. Thompson and A. E. Hedbeck, listed in the readings, provide minimal additional data.

The Result

1-15. Achenbaum, W. A. (1983). Shades of gray: Old age, American values, and federal policies since 1920. Boston: Little, Brown.

This book explores the reasons why current programs for the aged were developed and instituted. It discusses how recent American history and the policies of "modernization" have acted upon the lives of older people and the ways in which the elderly have adapted and coped with a changing society. The format of the book is conceptualized through a set of seven conflicting American values: (1) self-reliance vs. dependency, (2) expectation vs. entitlement, (3) work vs. leisure, (4) the individual vs. family, (5) private vs. public, (6) equity vs. adequacy, and (7) novelty vs. tradition. Achenbaum discusses the effect of these counter values on political forces within the society. The making of federal policy from the Great Depression through Reaganomics is examined in the context of the influence of these opposing values on the "watersheds" or important divisions in our national history. The conclusion reflects the title of the work. The proper balance between American values and federal policies designed to meet the needs of the aging and the aged will continue to be drawn in "shades of gray." There is little evidence that the impact of modern values has been recognized or considered in the formation of policies and programs for the aged. The book is a cornerstone in gerontological history in that it initiates comparisons between the development of a science and its influence on and by social history.

1-16. Birren, J. E., Cunningham, W. R., & Yamamoto, K. (1983). Psychology of adult development and aging. Annual Review of Psychology, 34, 543-575.

In this research article, the authors used two sources to examine literature and citations in the psychology of adult development and aging. First was an analysis of reviews in the *Annual Review of Psychology* across a span of thirty years, 1946-1975. Second, data bases were searched for relevant articles and books published between 1975 and 1981. These sources yielded more than 4000 articles related to the psychology of adulthood and aging. The results show an explosive growth in aging publications beginning in the 1960's, but this momentum lacked coherence, cross-references, and integration among the topics investigated. The authors conclude that psychological research moved forward through the study of particular behavioral processes or of a particular time in the lifespan with neither a theoretical base nor continuity. The breadth and depth of the article provide a sound historical review of past publications and a springboard to direct future attention to neglected topics of study.

1-17. Hoyer, W. J., Raskind, C. L., & Abrahams, J. P. (1984). Research practices in the psychology of aging: A survey of research published in the Journal of Gerontology, 1975-1982. Journal of Gerontology, 39, 44-48.

This is a follow-up of an earlier study by Abrahams et al. The authors summarize eight years (1975-1982) of research practices in the psychology of aging using 263 articles published in the Psychological Sciences Section of the *Journal of Gerontology*. Articles were examined for content, method of procedures and analysis, subject characteristics, and investigator characteristics. The authors determined the number and percentage of studies by content categories and years, the distribution of chronological ages of subjects, and percentage comparisons of health status, sex, data collection strategies, and statistical procedures. By using the results of this sample, they were able to point out neglected topics and the need for more specific data on the characteristics of subjects. Age limits were highly uneven; gender and health status were often not reported. Although the work covers only eight years of research in one aspect of aging, comparisons of the results and conclusions to the earlier Abrahams et al. study provide information on change across time and the current status of psychological research in aging.

1-18. Rasch, J. D. (1976). Institutional origins of articles in The Gerontologist: 1961-1975. The Gerontologist, 16, 276-279.

This work surveys the major articles published in the first fifteen years of *The Gerontologist* to determine the institutional origin of contributors. Its intent was to identify and give credit to institutions that have been major producers of gerontological literature. A total of 860 articles were identified. In cases of multiple authors with multiple institutional affiliations, credit for articles was proportionally divided. Results showed Duke University, the Veterans Administration, the University of Chicago, and the University of Southern California-Los Angeles to be the major contributors. Also prominent were the Philadelphia Geriatric Center and the University of California-Los Angeles. Although Rasch's results appear to be reliable, it is difficult to measure the many factors that contribute to a researcher's academic affiliation. Personal preferences and chance could easily influence the outcome of this research. The author does recognize the limitations of surveying only one journal and the problem of quantity versus significance.

1-19. Riegel, K. F. (1973). On the history of psychological gerontology. In C. Eisdorfer & M. P. Lawton (Eds.), The psychology of adult development and aging. Washington, DC: American Psychological Association.

This chapter discusses three historical aspects of aging. First, Riegel conducted a quantitative analysis of gerontological literature in psychology by retrieving citations for a root or "node" paper backwards across two generations to other articles and their citations. The study recorded 235 publications and a total number of 4,310 references. Second, the chapter focuses on underdeveloped areas of research. Third, the author concludes that the majority of studies in psychological aging are an enormous waste of effort expended on insignificant issues. The chapter offers far more than its intensive, comprehensive research and astute criticism of past shortcomings in the field. Through his research, Riegel is able to specify the areas of psychological gerontology that recapitulate and those in strong need of further investigation. He proceeds further to outline recommendations of criteria for knowledge in the field, goals in higher education, the use of technology, and a model of man and society that will direct studies in the psychology of gerontology toward their ultimate potential to alleviate problems in aging. The importance of this chapter cannot be overemphasized. It demonstrates the value of past history to a science; and, whether or not one agrees with Riegel that psychological research in aging is problematic beyond reform and must be revolutionized, his results and judgment merit serious consideration.

1-20. Seltzer, M. M. (1975). The quality of research is strained. The Gerontologist, 15, 503-507.

Seltzer examined and analyzed articles dealing with psychological processes, which were listed in Shock's *Current Publications in Gerontology and Geriatrics* published in the *Journal of Gerontology* in 1968. The criterion for inclusion was some type of psychological or social tests or measurements. Only forty-two of a total of 275 articles met this criterion. Within this sample, the author examined the characteristics of the samples and sampling frames, comparability of data, and issues of reliability and validity. Results of this analysis showed a disorder verging on chaos. Samples, operational definitions, and methods were not comparable. The author concludes that meta-research, research that investigates the nature of many data, is necessary if the science of gerontology is proceed in an orderly and cumulative manner. The article lays the groundwork for an advancement of scientific behavior in gerontology research and should be required reading for researchers in aging.

1-21. Shock, N. W. (1946-1980). Index of current publications in gerontology and geriatrics published in the Journal of Gerontology, Vols. 1-20.

This collected bibliography published in each of the above volumes of the *Journal of Gerontology* was begun and maintained by Nathan W. Shock. The Index is a veritable catalog of gerontological research from 1950 through 1980. Shock collected, read, and classified bibliographic items for all of the disciplines. His work provided a national and international contact among researchers in all aspects of aging. This outstanding effort and its results can serve as an historical record, a barometer in the measure of gerontological research across the years, and an index to the development of gerontology as a science.

2

INTERGENERATIONAL RELATIONSHIPS AND CAREGIVING

Mary Ann Kistner

INTRODUCTION

The early studies of intergenerational relationships and filial responsibility indicated that support for aging family members was being provided by kin and extended kin (Cicirelli, 1981; Robinson and Thurnher, 1979; Shanas, 1979). Since that time, intergenerational studies and caregiving literature have developed separate, although overlapping bodies of research. The intergenerational literature is concerned with generational and intergenerational interdependencies and the changing patterns of relationship which occur as the generations grow older (Bengtson, 1979; Cohler, 1983; Golan, 1988; Hagestad, 1986; Hess & Waring, 1978; Peterson, 1979; Troll & others, 1979). The caregiving literature, on the other hand, although concerned with patterns of relationship, addresses relationships where one individual is dependent upon the other for support; the care receiver is dependent upon assistance from a spouse, children, other kin, or friends (Archbold, 1983; Brody, 1983, 1990; Kaye & Applegate, 1990; Lang & Brody, 1983; Matthews & Rosner, 1988; Miller, 1987; Walker, 1991).

Moreover, much of the literature on caregiving is concerned with providing care for a cognitively impaired or cognitively and physically impaired individual which places greater demands for care on the caregiver than caring for an individual who is somewhat physically limited or impaired. Thus, even the caregiving literature is comprised of two main divisions: those studies of caregivers of the cognitively impaired and frailest elderly, and those of caregivers of the elderly with minor physical impairment who need some assistance.

The focus of this discussion will be primarily on the caregiving literature. Intergenerational studies have been included to clarify patterns of relationship in aging families so that any relationship changes brought about by the need for caregiving will be highlighted.   Additionally, much of the terminology which is used in the caregiving literature is explicated. in the intergenerational family literature, so the inclusion of this literature is important for basic understanding.

Caregiving has generated a huge body of research with a number of rather significant problems. One of the primary problems with the caregiving literature is that much of the research, primarily the earlier research, does not provide a definition for the term caregiver. Therefore, in many studies, the reader is uncertain whether the caregiver is providing instrumental and psychological/social care her/himself, or if she/he is purchasing instrumental care and providing primarily psychological and social support. Additionally, there has not been clarification in the studies as to whether the caregiver is the primary caregiver, a backup caregiver, or an occasional caregiver. There has also been a lack of clarification, in some cases, as to whether the caregiver is providing care for a care receiver who is living independently or is institutionalized. A whole body of research has been built upon a concept which was not clearly defined. Consequently, when comparing the findings of studies, the results are often ambiguous and not comparable because of the lack of clarity in definition.

Another problem was that until the later 1980s, there had been little attempt to use existing theoretical frameworks to guide studies, or to develop theory from the research completed. Much of the early caregiving literature has been descriptive and atheoretical. Researchers have focused on the effects of socioeconomic characteristics, who was providing care and how much, and whether there were any relationship or gender differences in the way that care was provided.   In the mid 1980s, the focus was on the definition, operationalization, and measurement of the burden of caregiving, particularly caregiving of the demented. At this time, a number of burden scales were developed. Research was done with purposive samples using caregivers who were in Alzheimer's support groups or were placing parents in nursing homes. Additionally, much of the research of that time utilized the secondary data from the National Long Term Care surveys of 1982 and 1984 and the National Long Term Care supplements. The samples used from these surveys were often of the frailest, most dependent elderly and the caregivers caring for them. Consequently, the literature has been "heavy" with studies of very dependent, frail care receivers, and very burdened caregivers.

As an outcome of this focus of research, in the late 1980s interest developed in looking at caregiving from a stress framework based on the model of Lazarus and Folkman. The stress orientation has continued to guide research into the 1990s and is important to caregiving literature. However, caregiving is also a family problem which often requires family decision making and co-operation. Some of the literature of the late 1980s and early 1990s is beginning to explore the dyadic relationship between caregiver and care receiver or a family orientation where care decisions are made and care is provided within a larger, extended family context. There is renewed interest in studying those persons who need and are dependent upon primarily physical assistance because they are "normatively" aging, rather than so heavily focusing on those who are cognitively impaired, or the frail elderly. Current renewed interest in normative caregiving will provide a more balanced view of caregiving in the aging population. Additionally, researchers are beginning to explore the benefits of caregiving as well as the costs using the Exchange framework. Studies are beginning to explore caregiving satisfaction in both caregiver and care receiver.

The articles reviewed in annotated form reflect the development of caregiving and intergenerational literature across time. Several articles were chosen because these are classics in caregiving and intergenerational literature (Hess & Waring, 1978; Shanas, 1979; Treas, 1977). Others were chosen because they are representative of a researcher who is particularly strong in a particular area (Bengtson, 1979; Brody, 1981, 1990; Cantor, 1983; Hagestad, 1986, 1988; Troll & others, 1979). Several articles were chosen because they reflect newer trends in the methodology or theoretical direction of research (Archbold, 1983; Brody and others, 1983; Johnson & Barer, 1990; Matthews & Rosner, 1988; Sheehan & Nuttall, 1988; Zarit & others, 1986). Other articles which are included but have not been cited in this essay were chosen because they are explanatory or fill in the gaps between the broad categories which have been mentioned. Overall, there is an interesting sampling of the literature which is representative of the caregiving/intergenerational literature available.

ANNOTATED BIBLIOGRAPHY

2-1.   Antonucci, T.C. & Akiyama, H. (1987). An examination of sex differences in social support among older men and women. Sex Roles, 17, 737-749.

This article reports a study of mid-life and older couples to determine if there are gender differences in either qualitative and/or quantitative support provided to elders. This study is based on the Support of Elderly, a national survey of older persons. The participants chosen at random agreed to participate in one-hour face-to-face interviews with trained interviewers. Persons were asked to diagram support networks and were questioned of quality and quantity of relationships. Findings indicate that women receive more support from children and friends while men rely almost exclusively on wives to provide support. Both sexes prefer to provide more support than they receive, and both also find the quality of support more important than quantity of support for well-being. Women report both statistically significant larger networks of support and the receipt of a greater amount of support. Men report greater marital satisfaction than women.

Appropriate statistics were used to interpret the findings which were displayed in tabular form. The findings are useful for understanding the differences between male and female social support in older populations, the effects of marital disruption/death upon the survivor, and the types of social support which might be missing or that the individual might utilize.

2-2.   Archbold, P.G. (1983). Impact of parent-caring on women. Family Relations, 32, 39-45.

Thirty white caregivers and their functionally impaired parents or parents-in-law were interviewed separately, were observed in their home settings, and were asked to complete the Older American Resources and Services Multidimensional Functional Assessment (OARS) questionnaire measuring functional status in 5 areas. Qualitative data were used to determine that two caregiving modalities were employed by the caregiving women: the care-manager who purchased care and managed the caring for the care receiver, and the care-provider who provided direct care to the care receiver herself.

Findings indicated that socioeconomic status (SES) was the determining factor in the choice of caregiving styles; managers had higher incomes, more education, and were more likely to be employed in career-type positions which provided sufficient financial resources to purchase services. The care-providers were less satisfied and experienced more conflict and stress in the caregiving role than care-managers who were able to spend less time fulfilling parental instrumental needs. Care-managers could focus on fulfilling the psychological and social needs of the parent in activities which both the care-manager and parent would enjoy. Both care-managers and care-providers experienced costs of caregiving expressed as difficulties in their marriages, in sibling relationships, and in loss of personal time. Overall, higher costs and fewer rewards were experienced by care-providers than by care-managers.

The important contribution of the article is clarification of the term of caregiver which is used in many different ways in caregiving literature. However, the presentation of data seems to be somewhat incomplete; tables would be helpful in summarizing the differences and similarities between the two groups. Additionally, not addressed in the article were differences between the two groups that might affect outcomes, such as length of time in caregiving, age of caregiver, and level of impairment of parent. However, both data collection and interpretation seem to be adequate to establish the caregiving categories and the characteristics of each. This is one of the earliest qualitative studies of caregiving which focuses on the subjective experience of the caregiver and care receiver as the source of data.

2-3. Bengtson, V.L. (1979). Research perspectives in intergenerational interaction. In Ragan, P.K. (Ed.), Aging Parents (pp. 37-57). Los Angeles: University of Southern California Press.

The author defines three important concepts for understanding intergenerational relationships: cohort effect, lineage effect, and period effect. The concepts provide a way to understand differing perceptions between the generations regarding the way that the world is viewed. In spite of differences in the generations, there is a continuity maintained within the family system. Although the emphasis has seemed to be on generational differences and discontinuity, research from the California Longitudinal Study of Three Generation Families indicates both similarities and differences in values between cohorts and even stronger similarities along lineage (intrafamily) lines, in spite of cohort differences.

A general finding of this study was that there is a greater perception of generational difference than actually exists, and that this perception varies with the age. The younger group sees more differences than really exist; youth perceive that these differences occur in other person's families and that his/her family is somehow unique in its similarities. Developmental agendas affecting autonomy and dependence affect generational perceptions as do the differences in life history of the generations. The final portion of the chapter addresses generational problems including role transition, autonomy and dependency, equitable exchange, and continuity and disruption, as well as addressing problem solving techniques that families may use in working with these issues.

This is an informative article addressing intergenerational issues within the family system and also including conceptual definition and explanation. The use of personal intergenerational family histories to illustrate concepts increases understanding. The conclusion of the article humanizes family relationships, addressing both normal conflicts as well as negotiations within the family. The article indicates that continuities and discontinuities exist within all intergenerational family systems.

2-4. Brody, E.M. (1981). Women in the middle and family help to older people. Gerontologist, 21, 471-480.

The changing roles of women and the extension of the lifespan are examined together with both implications for the family and for social policy. Based on several studies of women and their aging parents, as well as a study of granddaughters, mothers, and grandmothers, Brody shows that the delivery of caregiving services must provide a better mix between community and family. The "woman in the middle" is increasingly involved in employment outside the home, mainly through economic necessity. In addition, the middle generation is approaching retirement and anticipates time to pursue personal interests without child care burdens. Both of these changes in the adult child generation occur at a time when elderly parents are living into their eighties and need care. In spite of changes in attitudes, the caregiving role is primarily assumed by the daughter with role overload often an outcome. Social policy must reflect a family policy which supports and enhances the family caregiving role rather than maintaining the institutional or family (women caregiver) perspective which now prevails. The mix of in-home care, respite, day-care, family-allowances, etc. to support the varying and individualistic needs of the elderly must be developed.

The article defines the problems of families in a time of change, highlighting that attitudes change, but not necessarily the behaviors that correspond to these attitudes. The central focus of the discussion is a call for a new social policy to provide assistance to the middle generation caregiver. The concern is valid, but a way to manage the costs of the changes remains a problem facing governments at all levels. Continued education will increase awareness of the problem, but monetary solutions remain an obstacle.

2-5. Brody, E.M. (1990). Women in the Middle: Their Parent Care Years. New York: Springer Publishing Company.

The book examines the central role that women play in caring for elderly parents. It is organized in three main parts. The first section deals primarily with demographics of parent-caring and the effects on the caregiver: these are statistical findings. The second part of the book humanizes the statistics, exploring caregiving from the inside view of the women involved in the day-to-day tasks of providing care; the author includes qualitative dialogue for understanding. The final part examines the contradictions between parent caring and employment outside of the home, as well as explores the conditions under which caregivers and their families make decisions to institutionalize the parent. The final chapter of the book is a summary and also includes suggestions for future agendas.

A significant part of the book presents a picture of caregiving based on the experiences of a nucleus of women who are in the most demanding caregiving situations and have reached the point where they are forced to apply for institutionalization of the parent or parent-in-law. The subjects of this book are caregivers who have been most severely stressed, and the picture presented reflects this stress as well as their distress. Overall, the book is an excellent broad-based compilation of the available research on caregiving. It includes a strong agenda for social institutions as well as a challenge for the modification of the contracts which exist between men and women regarding family issues and work.

2-6. Brody, E.M., Johnson, P.T., Fulcomer, M.C., and Lang, A.M. (1983). Women's changing roles and help to elderly parents: Attitudes of three generations of women. Journal of Gerontology, 38, 597-607.

Concerns in this article focus on the impact of changing lifestyles and roles in the American family and the possible impact of these changes on the care of elderly family members. The declining birth rate, the increasing life span, and the increasing number of women in the labor market are important changes impacting on caregiving attitudes and behaviors. This study was based on a sample of 403 Philadelphia women, three generations, from 213 families; 75 triads were from the same three generation families and the remainder were members of three generation families which fit one of the three categories investigated, which were grandmother, mother, or adult granddaughter. The instrument used, although not specifically identified, focused on beliefs, action orientations, and feelings. The strategy of the research focused on relationships, and three hypotheses concerned with differences between egalitarian gender roles and responsibility toward aging parents were proposed. Findings indicated some differences between the generations regarding gender roles and caregiving, but also a high level of agreement. The findings which load primarily on five factors are presented in extensive tabular form.

The authors indicate that the sample is not representative of the population and that results cannot be generalized. The findings do, however, provide insights into attitudinal changes which have occurred across cohort lines regarding gender roles and generational familial responsibilities. The application of these findings for policy makers would be somewhat suspect, since the educational level of the middle and younger generations is quite high, and the level of employment of the women, particularly in the middle generation, is also very high. It, therefore, might be assumed that attitudes toward egalitarian roles in the middle generation might be higher than the norm. Also, because there is both a family related portion of the sample as well as a non-related portion, family transmitted values are not known and the combined sample confounds the effect of these results. In spite of these shortcomings, this is a significant study dealing with generational concerns and issues for women.

2-7. Cantor, M.H. (1983). Strain among caregivers: A study of experience in the United States. Gerontologist, 23, 597-604.

The study presented is part of a larger study of marginal income, frail elderly clients and their primary caregivers who are served by a homemaker service in New York City. This particular study involved 111 clients and their primary caregivers who would benefit from limited special services. These caregivers were identified as spouses, adult children, other relatives, or friends/neighbors. The findings of the study indicated that there were differences in the amount of strain experienced by caregivers which were directly related to closeness in the relationship bond; spouses exhibited the greatest strain and friends/neighbors the least. Additionally, contributing to strain were the degree of caregiver worry, familism, gender of caregiver, and relationship quality between caregiver and care receiver. Women were likely to experience greater strain than were men as caregivers. The article concludes with the types of support services most useful to each of the categories of caregivers, including combinations of care services and incentives.

Methodologically, this was a very complete, well-designed study with results clearly explained. In particular, all the statistical procedures used were presented and the results elaborated in the verbal portion of the article. The study provided evidence that primary caregivers are not a homogeneous group, and that the stress and strain of caregiving differs by gender as well as by the closeness of the bond between the primary caregiver and the care receiver. Overall, this study provided not only outcomes of the caregiving process, but also some potential solutions and policy suggestions which would have positive impact on each of the different types of caregivers.

2-8. Cicirelli, V.G. (1981). Helping Elderly Parents. Boston: Auburn House.

The book is the outcome of two studies completed by the author from a field survey of 164 adult children in Lafayette, Indiana who had at least one living parent over 60 years of age. One study is concerned with determining the needs of the elderly and how these are fulfilled by children. The second study and main thrust of this book is the response of adult children regarding their parent's needs, including the development of a model. The author uses existing theories to guide the study. The first theoretical focus is on attachment theory, the feeling that the child has for the parent which affects helping behaviors both in the present and in the future. Issues of ethnicity, class, age, sex, education, and other variables are considered to be included as part of attachment behaviors and are not addressed independently. The second theoretical perspective is stress effects which may impact upon the future commitment to help if the demands of the parent become too great. Although not contributing to the model, the author uses exchange theory for understanding some of the results.

This is a significant study of adult children/elderly parent relationships in a medium sized Midwestern city. The construction of the survey, the training of interviewers, and the method of data collection are appropriate for the broad based information. Having been grounded in a theoretical perspective also provides a focus for the findings of the study. The presentation of data and text is done very well; tables are embedded within the text to explain that particular data. It is important to note, however, that this study does not seem to include the old-old, or the frail elderly who provide an increased set of stresses above those mentioned in the book. Except for interactions with the old-old, this study provides insights for both generations so that the relationships between the two might be maintained with the least amount of stress possible.

2-9. Cicirelli, V.G. (1983). A comparison of helping behavior to elderly parents of adult children with intact and disrupted marriages. Gerontologist, 32, 619-625.

The study was a comparison of 141 adult children with disrupted marriages, (divorce, widowhood, and remarriage) and 164 adult children with intact marriages and the amount of support that is given to their elderly parents. There were no statistical differences in demographics between the two groups except that significantly more women from disrupted marriages were employed than women from intact marriages. The findings indicated that individuals from intact marriages gave significantly more help to their elderly parents than those with disrupted marriages. Additionally, children from disrupted marriages perceived their parent(s) as being less needy, felt that they had less obligation to their parents, and thought they had less time to help their parents because of job demands. In total help, there were statistically significant differences between the two groups, although overall the amount of help given by both was quite low. Using several other scales, the study indicates that the main reason for providing less help to parents in the disrupted group was the demands of job responsibilities.

The study was based on information gathered in 1980 and 1981 in field studies with, it may be assumed, a survey type instrument. Although the researcher tried to divide help into various subcategories in preliminary factor analysis, the questions formed only one factor. Additionally, the author addressed the issues of marital disruption and the changes that are brought about particularly because of changing economic needs. Practical suggestions for policy makers and practitioners are presented.

2-10. Cohler, B.J. (1983). Autonomy and interdependence in the family of adulthood: A psychological perspective. Gerontologist, 23, 33-39.

The author questions the more commonly held ideas regarding development that continue the intergenerational interdependence of the child and the mid-life parent into later life as a similar dependency between later life adult and adult-child. The author suggests that instead of interdependency being sought in later life, it is autonomy which is desired; the aging person needs to be freer to pursue his/her own needs. The development of attachment of the child for the mother as understood through social learning theory, ethology, and the psychoanalytic theories is useful, according to the author, for personality development through midlife, but at midlife there is discontinuity in personality; personality development becomes concerned with greater autonomy and interiority. The author cites other cultures where the person (he illustrates with only males) is able to withdraw from the interdependencies of business and family. In contrast to this autonomy, our culture focuses on the need to maintain and foster continuing relationships.

This perspective of later life development provokes a number of questions regarding the changing demographics of aging, particularly the growth of the old-old who seem to turn to their children for some support as their health begins to fail. The author cites the need for autonomy past mid-life and indicates that the intergenerational ties of children and grandchildren may be an intrusion on the desired roles for later life of the young-old. However, it seems there would need to be radical changes in social policy or in demographics so that the old-old, who eventually need health care support, will have assistance available without impinging on the autonomy of their young-old children. While the article examines intergenerational ties from later mid-life and interdependencies with the younger generations, it was not concerned with later mid-life and the older generation and the impact of the needs of the old-old on the potential for later autonomy of the young-old.

2-11. Dunham, C.D. & Bengtson, V.L. (1986). Conceptual and theoretical perspectives on generational relations. In Datan, N., Greene, A.L., & Reese, H.W. (Eds.), Life-Span Developmental Psychology (p. 1-27). Hillsdale, NJ: Lawrence Erlbaum Associates.

According to the authors, problems with research involving different generations and the resulting generational relationships indicate a need to utilize clearly defined concepts. Additionally, there is a need to link studies of intergenerational relationships within the broader theoretical frameworks of sociology and psychology. Based on these two ideas, the authors proceed to define and clarify seven important concepts. The first four are primary to generational relationships: generation, cohort, generation units seen as forerunners and keynoters (societal change agents) and cohort based social movements, and lineage. Three concepts are related to lineage levels of intergenerational interactions: norms, socialization, and solidarity. The intersects of these three concepts with cohort and lineage are important to intergenerational understanding. The two dimensions of historical and individual/developmental time and the micro and macro social dimensions add to the complexity. Theoretical frameworks helpful for studying intergenerational relationships are social conflict, functionalism, interactionism, social learning, and psychoanalytic.

This presentation identifies constructs and defines concepts which are useful for understanding intergenerational relationships and family interdependencies. Situations explicating the use of particular theoretical frameworks within the context of family issues provide potential intergenerational researchers a basic understanding of the theories presented. This is a good resource article for those interested in either pursuing or better understanding the complexities of intergenerational research.

2-12. Finley, N.J., Roberts M. D., & Banahan III, B.F. (1988). Motivators and inhibitors of attitudes of filial obligation toward aging parents. Gerontologist, 28, 73-78.

The variables which are thought to enhance filial obligation were examined to determine if the gender of the adult child and the gender of the parent or the parent-in-law makes a difference. Early data had shown mixed outcomes. Data for this study were obtained by telephone information from 667 persons who indicated having a parent over 70 years old and were willing to be interviewed. Demographics were assessed and several scales to measure affection and role conflict were employed. Multiple regression analysis was applied to data on each parent and parent-in-law. Differences in filial obligation between mother, father, mother-in-law, and father-in-law were found and these were gender dependent. Additionally, several demographic variables affected filial obligation such as race, number of siblings, education, and income. This study found that filial obligation is dependent on many things, most importantly the parent involved and the gender of the adult child.

The methodology of the study seemed appropriate and the findings supported those of other studies regarding parental and gender differences. However, the assumption that affection produces obligation, particularly in males, is challenged by the findings and requires further study. The effects of the other variables, particularly of role conflict in women, need to be understood better. Role conflict was found not to be a significant factor affecting obligation towards mothers for females, but was found to negatively affect women's obligations toward fathers. Other areas for further study are the effect of number of siblings, and male/father and female/mother-in law relationships. The study provokes a number of new areas for study.

2-13. Giordano, J.A. (1988). Parents of the baby boomers: A new generation of the young-old. Family Relations, 37, 411-414.

The article attempts to predict family relationships and life styles as the generation preceding the baby boomers moves toward retirement. Including an older generation of what may be called the old-old, four and even five generation families will become a more common occurrence. The author predicts demographic changes in marriage, divorce, and remarriage rates as well as changes in public policy will direct services for the elderly more towards the private sector; the focus will be to enhance the quality of life. According to the author, there will be greater variety in lifestyles and more self-determination in achieving them.

Much of what is written in the article is based on oversimplified generalization. Policy issues regarding public and private financing of health care and services focus primarily on private financing; additionally, the public is viewed as being informed consumers of these services. Near the end of this article, the author states that the information in the article pertains to middle class individuals, primarily, but the caveat comes late in the discussion. This article assumes a dualistic, simplistic stance and does not adequately address the issues that will become paramount when there are two generations of retired old in many families.

2-14. Golan, N. (1988). The Perilous Bridge: Helping clients through mid-life transition. New York: The Free Press.

The focus is on midlife and the two main changes which occur: the redefinition of relationships with children and the readjustment of the bonds with aging parents. During the life course of the middle aged parent, there has been an exchange of tangibles and intangibles with the aging parents, predominantly moving downward. At midlife, however, the exchange changes directions and the flow of goods and services begins to move upward to the aging parent. There is on the part of the parent an expectation of help, and depending upon class, ethnicity, religion, and perhaps other factors, the intensity of this help is defined. The acceptance of responsibility for concrete assistance is filial responsibility; another important concept is filial maturity, the recognition by the adult child that the parent is becoming dependent upon him/her and that assistance can be presented in a non-threatening way. The bond between the parent and the adult child becomes more strained as the child perceives that the parent is dependent upon him/her and is often further strained by the realization by the adult child of his/her own decreasing abilities and aging issues. The book presents a series of case studies illustrating parental dyadic changes, personalizing and intensifying midlife intergenerational issues.

The current research and conceptual issues confronting intergenerational researchers are presented in this book in case study format. This adds a strong human value, and the issues become much more personal. Although there are strong ethnic undertones to these cases, the concepts are clearly presented and issues illustrated. Of particular interest to the persons studying aged issues are the intergenerational articles focusing on middle age relationships and the elderly.

2-15. Hagestad, G.O. (1986). The aging society as a context for family life. Daedalus, 115, 119-139.

In this article, Hagestad provides a critical review of patterns of family relationships within the context of an aging society. The lengthening of the life span has made common four and five generational families in which two generations may be classified as old. Existing role patterns are being challenged and new norms have not yet been established. Interdependencies which were previously economically necessary have become voluntary because of changes in social policy. Women seem to retain strong vertical ties with family (ties with both older and younger generations) while men maintain horizontal ties (ties with those of their generation). The duration of life, particularly for women, and the patterns of marital stability have had a profound effect upon family life. Women's aging and men's aging may continue to develop into very different experiences based on divorce and marriage patterns as well as patterns of remarriage.

The article is a good overview of existing research. It is not overly comprehensive in any area, but incorporates findings into an analysis of trends which are occurring in family relationships and in family structure and patterns. Important demographic changes are reviewed, discussed, and placed within the context of the 21st century family. This is a good basic article for understanding the effects of changing demographics upon the extended family.

2-16. Hagestad, G.O. (1988). Demographic change and the life course: Some emerging trends in the family. Family Relations, 37, 405-410.

The demographics of the family have changed considerably affecting the prevalence and timing of key family transitions. Death is more predictable, as is grandparenthood. The years of childbearing are more confined, and there is a more distinctive mark between generations. Divorce and remarriage have caused countertransitions in two generations: children and parents. In particular, divorce has had a profound influence on changing the children's life course. Remarriage, too, brings new step-siblings, step-grandparents, step-parents; there is a complicated web of new relationships with which to interact. There are also strong indications that off-time transitions present complications and problems throughout this web. These webs of relationships are extremely complex as the extension of the life span increases the layering effect of generations.

The author briefly examines the impact of these changing demographics on families and indicates that research in many areas is non-existent or incomplete. For example, the effects of divorce on adult children, in particular, and on aging parents are areas in which there is almost no research. The article calls for research in new areas to provide better understanding of family interrelationships. It also indicates the complexity of this type of research and the new direction in which family research must begin to move.

2-17. Hess, B.B. & Waring, J.M. (1978). Changing patterns of aging and family bonds in later life. Family Coordinator, 27, 303-314.

This is a review of demographic trends and the research literature supporting intergenerational bonding. Based on cohort differences, Hess and Waring predict that future elderly and their adult children will be quite different than the older and middle generations are now. As a cohort the older generation will be more educated, more financially independent, and better equipped to survive for a considerable time together as a couple without assistance from children. Norms regarding expected behaviors are changing, too, and there is more freedom for both men and women from previous stereotypes. As a result of these changes and many others, the bonds between the generations will become much more voluntaristic than they have ever been.

This is an excellent comprehensive overview of the literature from the life course perspective. Concern is not only with the life course in general, but changes which have occurred in demographics through succeeding cohorts. There is emphasis on the impact of the intersections of the elderly and their adult children for the elderly near the end of the life course. Projections of future intergenerational change are made based on changes in economics, health, roles, and many other variables which will impact upon and be caused by these cohorts as they move through time.

2-18. Johnson, C.L. (1988). Postdivorce reorganization of relationships between divorcing children and their parents. Journal of Marriage and the Family, 50, 221-231.

This is a longitudinal study of 40 months which examines the reorganization patterns of relationships of the adult child, particularly the relationships with aging parents, after divorce. Three different groups were established. The first group, the Generationals, were equally divided between males and females, were socially and financially dependent on parents, viewed the former spouse with hostility, had limited contact with in-laws, maintained more traditional moral values, and rarely cohabited or remarried. The second group, the Nucleated, were equally divided by gender, maintained firm boundaries around their primary family, received less economic and social support from families, established a more neutral relationship with the ex-spouse, maintained traditional values regarding morality, and more often remarried. The third group, 75% women and 25% men, were called the Network group; they were very individualistic, often retained strong relationships with in-laws, maintained friendly relationships with ex-spouses, maintained distance with their family of origin, were less dependent economically on parents, were less traditional in moral values, and more often remarried or cohabited. The process of divorce readjustment was described to be dynamic and intense. In quantitative measurements, these differences were not as significant as the researchers found them to be qualitatively.

The methodology of the study was very interesting, but there were significant variable problems which may have confounded results. The length of marriage and/or age of the divorcing adult was not considered, nor was the prior relationship of the adult with his/her parents. Therefore, one is uncertain whether the patterns which existed at 40 months were a continuation of patterns of adult child/parent relationships that had existed before the divorce. Also, individuals over 45 or 50 with long term marriages might have different dependency relationships with their parents than those individuals who were younger or in shorter term marriages. These two areas, in particular, would be important for further study for understanding both the immediate effect and the long term effect of reorganization after divorce and the impact upon intergenerational relationships.

2-19. Johnson, C.L. & Barer, B.M. (1990). Families and networks among older inner-city Blacks. Gerontologist, 30, 726-733.

The study was concerned with the composition and functioning of social networks in the lives of elderly, inner-city blacks of low socioeconomic status (SES). Additionally, the black sample was compared with whites of the same SES and inner city location, to indicate differences which exist that are racially based. There were some differences in demographic variables between whites and blacks, but levels of perceived health, uses of formal support, and levels of functional impairment were comparable between the two groups.

This study, which was part of a larger research program, employed both quantitative and qualitative methodology. Focused interviews were done with a white sample of 52 and a black sample of 129; after one year 43% of the black sample was reinterviewed for further data collection regarding family process and kinship relationships. Findings indicated that relatives provided statistically more instrumental support to blacks than relatives did to whites. Additionally, in black networks, children, relatives, and friends provided more emotional support than did the same networks to whites. Central to more than 50% of black women's lives was the church. In black families, family relationships, although important, were independent and a high level of interdependency was not expected or achieved. Fictive kin were as likely as family to provide emotional support, and sibling relationships were important where siblings existed. The main difference in networks between blacks and whites was that blacks maintain a more extensive friendship and associational network than do whites. The relationships for blacks were dynamic, flexible, and changing within the family and extended family structure, and these patterns are functional for the elderly to maintain support where family is either unwilling or unable to assist.

A deficiency of the study was that a follow-up study was not done with a white subsample, so pattern changes which may have occurred in whites over time may have been missed or excluded. In general, the outcomes of the study support findings of other researchers studying black family patterns helping to unravel the confounding between race and SES. Clearly, the study indicates that there are racial differences between blacks and whites in social networks which are not the result of differences in SES.

2-20. Johnson, E. S. & Bursk, B.J. (1977). Relationships between the elderly and their adult children. Gerontologist, 17, 90-96.

The study examines the affective quality of relationships between aging white, elderly parents and their adult children on four indicators thought to affect relationships: health, finances, attitudes toward aging, and living environments. Additionally, there were questions involving family relationships and satisfaction. A structured interview schedule with both open ended and closed questions was prepared for both the parent group and the adult children group. Findings from both instruments indicated that attitudes toward aging and health were the most important correlates of the affective quality and the family relationship indicator. Using multiple regression analysis, about 25% of the variance was accounted for by the four variables. When parent's rating of the relationship was analyzed, the perception of parent's adequacy of income was the most important variable; the more positively perceived that income was, the more positively perceived was the parent-child relationship. The authors present several trends or themes within the four life areas which were obtained from their data. The article concludes with the import of effective health care for the elderly and support for the adult children to maintain quality caring relationships.

The article consisted of an extensive overview of the literature regarding the relationships between older people and their adult children. The methodology of the study seemed appropriate for gathering information, and statistical analysis provided both parent and parent/child information. Missing, though, was any presentation of data collected as part of the surveys and findings; this made it difficult to follow the correlations between variables as well as the regression factors. Presentation in tabular form would have made the data much easier to read and to understand.

2-21. Kaye, L.W. & Applegate, J.S. (1990). Men as elder caregivers: A response to changing families. <u>American Journal of Orthopsychiatry</u>, <u>60</u>, 86-94.

This study is part of a larger study based on a mail survey of 148 men who were part of caregiver support groups in the United States. The main purpose of the survey was to gather baseline data in a number of areas including gender-orientation of the male caregivers, the focus of this particular study. The majority of the care receivers were wives of the caregivers suffering from Alzheimer's Disease or other related disorders. Using the Sex Role Index (SRI), it was found that the caregiving men viewed themselves as fairly androgynous, possessing both instrumental and affective traits. Correlations between affective and instrumental trait factors were performed with a number of other variables. Findings, in general, indicated that men who were more instrumentally oriented were more satisfied with the caregiving role, viewed themselves as competent, and initiated affective behavior. Men who were more affectively oriented perceived less caregiving burden, were equally competent to the more instrumental men, initiated affective behavior more often than more instrumental men, and were affiliative. Overall, according to the authors, male caregivers saw their primary task as providing social support.

The methodology of the study, including the definition of caregiving, lacked clarity. There was no indication if these men were the only caregivers, or primary caregivers, nor of how much formal support was used within the household. Additionally, the authors described the men as androgynous, but then developed affective and instrumental typologies with no presentation of how many men were of each typology. A table presented an overall affective-instrumental profile of the sample, but not the different profiles for the two typologies. Overall, the study was lacking in direction and did not fulfill the expectation of providing information regarding men as caregivers of mentally impaired elders. Finally, the sample was of higher socioeconomic status (SES) as a group than the general population and all were white.

2-22. Lang, A.M. & Brody, E.M. (1983). Characteristics of middle-aged daughters and help to their elderly mothers. <u>Journal of Marriage and the Family</u>, <u>45</u>, 193-202.

The study focuses on the middle generation as providers of care for aging mothers. Issues of amount of time spent in caring and the types of care given are examined in regard to the living arrangement of the daughter (with mother or not), marital status (married or not), work status (employed or not), and age of caregiver (40-49 or 50 +). Findings indicate that the most assistance comes from daughters who live in the same household as the mothers, and that age has a significant effect upon the amount of help given. These two factors, residence and age, account for almost 38% of the variance in the hours of help provided. Work and marital status each account for an additional 2% of the variance; those who work and those who are married spend slightly less time providing assistance to mothers than do those who are unmarried and/or unemployed.

The sample for the study was small, urban, and non-representative of the general population. Data were collected by trained female interviewers in the subject's homes using a precoded interview schedule. Most of the statistical data is descriptive, but one-way analysis of variance (Anova) was used to compare each of the independent variables with the dependent variable (amount of help provided). The authors indicate that many of the findings obtained from this study are confirmatory of other studies performed on larger national sample data sets. However, the study also points to the need to know more of the effects of different marital status, as well as the effects of professionalization of jobs and the time involvement of employment, part-time or full-time.

2-23. Matthews, S. H., & Rosner, T. T. (1988). Shared filial responsibility: The family as the primary caregiver. Journal of Marriage & the Family, 50, 185-195.

The article examines the organization of older siblings to fulfill the needs of their aging parents. This is a preliminary study involving 50 sibling/family groups. Each group had at least two sisters who agreed to be interviewed, one employed, the other not employed outside the home. At least one parent was 75 or older; in only 12 of the families were both parents living and together. Data were gathered through a written questionnaire and follow up either in-person or by phone interview, with different persons interviewing each sister. Analysis was qualitative.

Five styles of participation were identified: routine, backup, circumscribed, sporadic, and dissociation. The styles of the siblings were often dictated by their employment, the support or not of the sibling's spouse, the proximity of the parent, the roles that the siblings have assumed in the family, the number of siblings in the family, and the gender of the siblings. Routine and backup participation were mostly provided by women, while either males or females were sporadic, disassociated, or circumscribed participants. Where there were only two female siblings, both were usually involved as caretaker or as caretaker and the backup; a greater number of siblings allowed for more diversity of styles. Whether siblings relationships were good or not, siblings came together to support parent's needs. Support levels were discussed among siblings and the unstated principle of least involvement was generally adopted to allow the parent(s) the highest level of independence. As needs became greater, additional help was often bought and paid for with the parent's monies.

The methodology seemed appropriate, and interesting results depict the ties that the adult siblings have with each other and with the parents based on the roles and ties that have continued throughout family development. The focus, too, places caregiving within the family structure rather than on a single family member. The study is identified as preliminary by the authors and weaknesses and deficiencies are specified.

2-24. Miller, B. (1987). Gender and control among spouses of the cognitively impaired: A research note. Gerontologist, 27, 447-453.

Fifteen middle-class white caregivers, nine women and six men, with cognitively impaired spouses comprised the sample. Most caregivers had known of the cognitive impairment for at least three years; two were more recent diagnoses. Using a semi-structured interview, the caregivers were questioned regarding patient care, changes in their lives, and barriers in care provision occurring since their spouses became impaired. Findings indicated that differences in caregiving were not attributable to level of impairment, but rather to different perceptions of both the impairment and the caregiving role. For women caregivers, changes in relationship brought about by the impairment were more difficult to accept. Men were more able to assume authority and control while continuing to pursue their own interests. Men were also more likely to be the only caregiver while women more often purchased help. Children provided emotional support but very little instrumental help. Relationships with friends changed over time as the spouse became more impaired. In general, there were gender differences in the management of the impaired spouse with men exhibiting less emotional stress than women.

A deficiency in the study was the smaller sample of husbands, and the extreme differences in their age range, from 60 to 89, a much different sample group than the wives who were all in their middle sixties and seventies; these age differences may have an impact on the outcomes of the study. This study, however, supports findings of other studies which note gender differences in both stress and burden associated with the caregiving role. Additionally, the study provides understanding of the differences in the interpretation of the disease process, the way that authority is assumed, the manner in which space and time are controlled, and the uses of both formal and informal social supports.

2-25. Peterson, J.A. (1979). The relationships of middle-aged children and their parents. In Ragan, P.K. (Ed.), Aging Parents (pp. 27-36). Los Angeles: University of Southern California Press.

Intergenerational relationships vary in closeness dependent upon the stages in the family life span. In this chapter, the relationships of middle-aged children and their aging parents are explored, and there is discussion of what is currently known from research about each of these generations as well as their interactions. The article also addresses the myths and unknown areas of generational relationships. Most generally, the author concludes that there are many differences based on ethnicity and economics, in particular, which define relationships between the generational groups.

The chapter is a general overview of relationships between children and parents at various stages in the life cycle. Some personal family insights are presented to illustrate the research data incorporated into the chapter. The author also comments on the differences between the more hedonistic pre-adolescents and adolescents of the 1960s and those adolescents in earlier cohorts in conjunction with the intergenerational changes which may or may not have occurred.

2-26. Pruchno, R.A., Blow, F.C. & Smyer, M.A. (1984). Life events and interdependent lives: Implications for research and intervention. Human Development, 27, 31-41.

The focus of the article is on the importance of the life web as both a unit of research and of intervention. From this perspective, an event which affects an individual has an impact beyond the individual and causes changes for those who share membership in that life web. An individual may hold membership in many webs, some of them fairly constant through the life course, and other webs which may change. For instance, the authors discuss divorce in mid/later life and its impact on the older parent generation as well as on the younger generation(s) of the family web. Intervention for these stressors would be most effective if it was intergenerational and encompassed those within the web. Additionally, it would be important to study the impact of several concurrent life stressors on a network (a group of webs in which a person has membership) and the differential effect(s) on the members.

This is an interesting article presenting the complexities of research models which cannot be interpreted unidimensionally, but which must be developed to study families in a new way. Not only is the focus of analysis changed from the individual to the family level, but the focus of intervention changes to a more complex level demanding new models and modes of intervention. The inclusion of greater numbers of subjects in both study and intervention has the potential to cause problems, both in definition and methodology. It would seem that it would be important to set achievable parameters, or research would begin to extend into webs of webs, etc., approaching a level of chaos. On the other hand, it is important to study the family beyond the level of the individual or even the nuclear family to that of multigenerational extended families.

2-27. Quinn, W.H. (1983). Personal and family adjustment in later life. Journal of Marriage and the Family, 45, 57-73.

The author used existing literature on intergenerational relationships to review variables which had been found to contribute to intergenerational well-being. Using several established and tested scales and measures, the author tested 143 parent-adult dyads to measure the 15 identified variables. Prior to the testing, a path model based on the research data was proposed. Findings indicated that 36.4% of the variance of psychological well being of the older parent was attributable to the parent's health. The second strongest predictor of parental psychological well being was the quality of the parent-child relationship, which was influenced by both affection and communication. A revised path model based on the findings of the study was proposed for future consideration and testing.

There are some difficulties with the methodology of the study. The author clearly indicates sampling processes, but there is a lack of clarity as to whether the sample is representative of the general population or of the southeastern city in which the study was done. Also, to study fifteen independent variables, a sample size of 143 parent-child dyads is quite small, although within an acceptable range. The statistical procedures followed by the author were not clearly explained, and it is difficult for the reader to follow the research data presented. Additionally, the results which are obtained are not very clear.

2-28. Robinson, B. & Thurnher, M. (1979). Taking care of aged parents: A family cycle transition. Gerontologist, 19, 586-593.

This study was based on a sample of adult children and parents who were part of a larger, longitudinal study of five year duration assessing psychological and social changes over the life course. This sample of 49 was interviewed using an open-ended instrument. Findings indicated that children felt a strong sense of obligation for their parent's care and well-being. Where parents were most dependent, the parent/adult child relationship was most difficult. Strong, positive relationships between the parent and the child were more likely when parents had active, busy lives of their own. Many of these adult children experienced a great deal of guilt regarding what they should do for their parents and performed tasks at great expense to their own health and well-being. Over the time of the study, several parents were placed in long term care facilities, while others who had lived independently took up residence in their child's home. Mental deterioration of the parent was stress producing, as was the perception by adult children that their parent(s) were restricting their lives and taking the freedom that they had "earned" in raising their families.

The parent-child relationships were assessed over three interview times. The dynamics and the intricacies of the relationship were expressed, and the interdependencies revealed. Findings of this study were supportive of quantitative studies that indicated a need for changes in policy to provide respite care for the caretaker and/or household care for the elderly when the burden on the caretaker became extreme. Support might serve as a deterrent in relationship deterioration between the generations. Additionally, caretaking children need to be aware of services available so that they might obtain needed relief.

2-29. Shanas, E. (1979). Social myth as hypothesis: The case of the family relations of old people. Gerontologist, 19, 3-9.

Concerns with aging and the involvement of family members in the aging process, including the myth that families do not care for the elderly, are briefly addressed. Additionally, the definitions of family as related kin, either through blood or through marriage, and household as those persons who act as though related or are related who live under the same roof are clarified; these terms have presented conceptual confusion and have contributed to a lack of clarity in research. The data are drawn from nationwide probability samples from 1957, 1962, and 1975. The findings present both constancies and changes which have occurred in families over the 18 year time period. In general, parents were no more distant in proximity from their children in the late 1970s then they were in the late 1950s, in spite of increases in geographic mobility. Additionally, there seems to be no less frequency of visiting between parents and their adult children than in the 1950s, and the number of parents who do not see their children frequently has remained stable. Even though children are important to the elderly, frequent contact with siblings and other relatives is also maintained. The final finding from the survey was that even with the addition of Medicare in 1966, from 1962 to 1975 there was no significant change in either the number of bedfast elderly being taken care of at home nor in those who have no relatives and have been institutionalized. In general, elderly with families are put in institutions as a last resort, after all other avenues have been exhausted.

The article is a well-written, well-presented view of what may be generalized over a twenty year period regarding family patterns of care of the aging, including a discussion of the need for conceptual clarity. Although presenting little new information, this is an excellent summary from survey data at three different points in time. Additionally, the conclusion provides the reader with directions for further research both with family relationships and with social policy to impact on the elderly and their families. This is one of the early classic articles regarding the intergenerational relationships of caring between adult children and their aging parents.

2-30. Shanas, E. (1979). The family as a social support system in old age. Gerontologist, 19, 169-174.

The study uses the data of a national survey of non-institutionalized persons who were 65 or older at the time of collection in 1975. The data were interpreted in two areas: family care for the elderly and family visiting patterns. Findings indicate that family and extended kin provide the major support to the elderly in need of assistance. If the spouse is alive, he/she provides the most help. Other help comes from children, or primarily from children if there is no spouse. Some help may be purchased. Frequent visiting and contact takes place, particularly with children. For those persons who are childless, contact with siblings becomes more frequent. Agency support is not sought, it seems, until other sources have been exhausted.

The article presents data which is applicable with a high confidence level to the general population since sampling was carefully controlled. This is a good basic article, but it may have become somewhat dated since there have been significant agency policy decisions made in the past 15 years which impact on family support, in general. However, the findings do indicate that family support and contact are high, and family support is the most desired support.

2-31. Sheehan, N.W. & Nuttall, P. (1988). Conflict, emotion, and personal strain among family caregivers. Family Relations, 37, 92-98.

The sample for this study was a mixed-age group of 98 family caregivers, about 75% of whom were caring for an elderly parent or parent-in-law and 25% who were caring for spouses. Over 80% of the sample was female. All completed self-administered questionnaires on demographics, the activities of daily living (ADL) checklist on functional impairment, the Memory and Behavior Problems Checklist, The Hopkins Symptoms Checklist, and scales on affection and satisfaction with caregiving, interpersonal conflict, personal strain, and negative emotion. Data were analyzed using the Pearson correlation and stepwise multiple regression methods. Findings are presented regarding a number of variables and their relationship with strain and with negative emotions. Additionally, data from the Hopkins Symptoms Checklist was used to compare depression, anxiety, and somatization with both negative emotion and strain, as well as other assessed variables. Of significance was the importance of subjective factors in regard to the consequences of caregiving.

This was one of few studies which assessed satisfaction with the caregiving role.

There was a significant amount of data generated in the study and the findings were clearly discussed and presented in tabular form. The article presented implications for practitioners, particularly in regard to the importance of the negative impact of conflict and its effects on caregivers' lives. There were also programs and models suggested to address stress and conflict within the lives of caregivers. This is a very comprehensive study.

2-32. Spitze, G. & Logan, J. (1989). Gender differences in family support: Is there a payoff? Gerontologist, 29, 108-113.

The study explores whether women receive more help and assistance in old age than men, particularly since women have devoted more time and energy to kinkeeping activities earlier in the life cycle. Is there an obligation created through caregiving of the offspring as children that provides women with greater help and assistance, a payoff, in older years? Findings suggest that women do receive slightly more assistance than men at comparable age and marital status. However, women also have greater need for assistance, according to this study which is based on a large national survey, the supplement to the National Health Interview Survey.

The survey does not indicate quality of interaction between the parent and child either in earlier years when the child was young nor in later years when the parent was older. Though only weakly indicative of additional help based on gender, the findings do indicate that gender does affect distance from children, frequency of phone calls, and frequency of contact in the unmarried parent, while age differences have little effect. It would seem, however, that the study does little to advance the question of whether an exchange deficit accumulated by the woman allows the woman to "collect" this debt. Additionally, the study does not examine exchange surplus that may be generated by men based on other factors than kinkeeping activities that might also have the effect of building a deficit. Although the study provided significant data, perhaps the hypothesis generated did not provide the best utilization of the data set.

2-33. Stueve, A., & O'Donnell, L. (1984). The daughter of aging parents. In Baruch, G., & Brooks-Gunn, J. (Eds.), Women in midlife (pp.203-225). New York: Plenum Press.

Parents and their adult children are sharing a longer span of time in which both are adults and also an extended time when the offspring provide help to their aging parents. The article primarily is concerned with two issues: 1) how adult children experience the long period when their parents are relatively healthy, and 2) how these children look at their commitment to their elderly parents. This study of 81 daughters of elderly parents examines the way that women of different social and life cycle positions interpret and frame the adult daughter role, taking into account increased opportunities in the labor force and the traditional commitment of women to assume the role of kinkeeper. Women may be at very different points in their own family or personal life cycles which involve different role commitments that, in turn, impact upon relationships with parents. Findings indicate working class daughters have closer and more interdependent relationships with parents than middle class women, who have stronger boundaries with their families of procreation and greater separation from the lives of their parents. Working class women provide more direct care to their parent(s) while middle class women purchase more care.

The sample chosen and the analysis done by the authors indicate that women with 70 year old parents are not a uniform group who are experiencing their parent's aging in the same way at the same point in their lives. More dialogue from the subjects would have been helpful to support the suggestions and conclusions which the authors make, but limitations of space make this difficult. Many finding from the qualitative study are supported by other research studies and these are cited; also, new areas of research as outcomes of this study are presented.

2-34. Treas, J. (1977). Family support system for the aged: Some social and demographic considerations. Gerontologist, 17, 486-491.

The author outlines the changes in the meaning of intergenerational support as the basis for support moved from the economic ties that parents held over their children to the affectional bonds which maintain support of the older generation by their offspring today. Changing demographics indicate fewer children to support parents; a change in employment patterns for women, both for economic necessity as well as self-fulfillment; and increased longevity of older adults. The interaction of these factors presents the need for evolving intergenerational relationships and social policies for caretaking of the aged. The author suggests monetary payments to those family members who provide the same services as nursing homes in a more personal, affectional way in their own homes. This is viewed as a possible way of addressing these social and demographic changes.

This classic article presents a good overview of the historical changes which have occurred in intergenerational relations over the past several centuries and makes recommendations for new policies based on the demographic projections for the next several decades. The article provides a framework for understanding intergenerational trends.

2-35. Troll, L.E., Miller, S.J., & Atchley, R.C. (1979). <u>Families in later life</u>. Belmont, CA: Wadsworth Publishing Company, Inc.

The authors take the perspective that the modified extended family is most important in understanding families in later life. The extensive research study data on families referred to in the book is cross sectional, so the changes over time which occur in the quality and quantity of relationships as well as the continuities and discontinuities of the extended family are not addressed. However, these long term bonds do exist and based on their own history establish patterns for the types of interaction which occur. The book addresses conceptual issues which affect the study of the family. An intergenerational developmental model based on the interaction of the individuals as well as the generations is assumed by the authors for this study. The topics which are addressed are older couples, being unmarried in later life, parents and their adult children, being a grandparent or great-grandparent, and siblings and kin. Statistical and demographic changes as well as common patterns in each of the topics are addressed. The book ends with the problems associated with the well being of older family members and their kin that might be addressed by policy makers.

This is a compilation of research on families and intergenerational patterns available at the time that it was written. The text provides a good overview of aging family patterns which are extensions of the traditional, nuclear family form. The snapshots of the family interactions are very general in nature and address issues more typical of the white, middle to upper-middle class family. The authors assume that most families fall into the structure that they have indicated and that interactions of the older family are based on this family form. There is only a minimal amount of recognition of working class families and issues of racial differences in spite of the fact that these are acknowledged as being important. Non-white, non-middle class families are only superficially addressed.

2-36. Walker, A.J. & Allen, K.R. (1991). Relationships between caregiving daughters and their elderly mothers. <u>Gerontologist</u>, <u>31</u>, 389-396.

The article focuses on the costs and rewards of caregiving based on the analysis of interview data of 29 pairs of widowed mothers and their primary caregiver daughters. The sample of care receivers was neither cognitively impaired nor severely functionally limited; care was provided in mainly instrumental tasks of daily living and in some personal care. Data were collected in face-to-face, semi-open interviews regarding the mothers health, the activities performed by the daughters, the caregiving situation itself, and the relationship between the members of the dyad. Data were analyzed for themes and patterns in the relationship which focused on positive and negative outcomes, concerns with the partner's outcomes, and the presence or absence of conflict. Three typologies of caregiving relationships emerged from the data based on the results of combined exchange within the dyad. Additionally, demographic differences within each of the groups indicated that the length of caregiving and the number of children of the caregiver affect satisfaction and conflict within the relationship. In contrast, the level of impairment did not affect satisfaction.

This study is somewhat unique for caregiving literature in that it is theoretically based on the exchange and conflict frameworks and that it considers the joint outcomes of the members of the caring dyad. Additionally, this is one of a small number of studies which assess benefits to the caregiver as an outcome of the caregiving experience. The methodology was explained in adequate detail with some explanation of both data analysis and coding methods. Although there was some attempt to elaborate demographic differences within the typologies, there was not an effort made to assess whether the relationship prior to the caregiving experience was a continuation of a formerly existing relationship pattern within the dyad. Overall, this was an interesting, informative study with the potential to generate further studies from a dyadic perspective rather than only from the perspective of the caregiver.

2-37. Weishaus, S. (1979). Aging is a family affair. In Ragan, P.K. (Ed.), Aging Parents (pp.154-174). Los Angeles: University of Southern California Press.

Issues of family relationships with the elderly were investigated with an elderly spouse, with aging siblings, and with adult children. Dependency relationships or mutual dependency relationships with a spouse seem to be of primary importance while relationships with siblings, particularly for those who have never married or have no children, increase in importance as the person ages. In contrast, there is a reluctance to intrude on children's lives. The relationships with children are extremely varied, with affection and frequency of interaction often not related. Generally, however, there is a recognition by children of a responsibility for their parent's emotional needs and an attempt to satisfy these. Parents tend to view relationships with children more positively than children view these relationships. Additionally, the literature in areas of parental morale, parent-child communication, childhood-parental/adult-parental feeling association, and mother-daughter relationship importance were presented and summarized. The chapter concluded with some clinical findings from a counseling group for middle-aged women who are experiencing difficulties with their older mothers, and the clinical explanations for these relationship problems. The article is a good overview of the changes in family relationships which occur with aging.   Of particular significance are the repeated themes of interdependency between spouses, among siblings, or among adult children and their parents.   The explanation of the therapeutic findings as well as some generalized goals for daughters are useful for women who are struggling with their relationships with their older mothers.   This is a very informative, helpful chapter for both persons with aging parents and students.

2-38.   Zarit, S.H., Todd, P.A. & Zarit, J.M. (1986). Subjective burden of husbands and wives as caregivers: A longitudinal study. Gerontologist, 26, 260-266.

This study was a two year follow-up of an earlier study on the experience of burden of 64 caregivers who were caring for a spouse with senile dementia. This study used the same measures as the previous study: the Zarit Burden Interview, the Mental Status Questionnaire (MSQ), the Face-Hand Test, the Zarit Memory and Behavior Problem Checklist, a social support scale, and a marital quality measurement.   Additionally, those who had institutionalized their spouses were asked additional questions regarding the placement decision. Findings at time 1 (T1) had indicated gender differences in burden and also strong evidence that subjective factors were more important in experienced burden than was the severity of the illness.   At time 2 (T2), findings indicate that the feeling of burden is associated with nursing home placement while the severity of symptoms is not primary to the placement decision.   Over time the caregiver's tolerance for problem behaviors increased; caregivers were able to establish routines which were not extremely burdensome.   Additionally, gender differences which had occurred at T1 were no longer present at T2, indicating that there may have been changes in the way that women coped.

The methodology of the study, the actual design and implementation, seemed adequate to address the issues of the study.   However, there are some sampling difficulties and definition problems.   The term caregiver is used, but the study does not clarify whether the spouse is the primary and only caregiver or a care manager.   Additionally, the sample was drawn from either a clinic which offered counseling and support groups or from an Alzheimer's Disease Advocacy group, but there is no indication in the study of the benefits that must result from the participation in these groups over the time that the caregiver participates in them.   Lacking is a baseline, i.e., either a time when the individual entered the supportive group, or a time when the experienced burden became great enough to require counseling and support.   The conclusions based on time are somewhat questionable.   Of significance, however is the confirmation that perceived burden is more important than actual impairment in the decision making process to institutionalize.   This study is very important in caregiving literature because of the longitudinal design, but is limited by the previously mentioned factors.

3

DECISION-MAKING RELATED TO HEALTH CARE AMONG THE ELDERLY

Kristin A. Thomas

INTRODUCTION

How do older persons become involved in decisions about their own health care? What are the roles of physician and family caregivers as either sources of information or decision makers when extent and type of medical treatment is addressed? This chapter addresses a range of readings that deal with a number of issues revolving around those questions. The chapter after this one focuses more directly on Do-not-resuscitate (DNR) orders.

One basic focus of several articles is the issue of the capacity or competence of elderly to make their own health care decisions. Diamond et al. (1989), Fitten et al. (1990), and Wettle et al. (1988) show that nursing home patients can be reliably categorized into those with the requisite capacity and those without. However, accuracy of physician judgments about capacity to decide was relatively low. Lo (1990) and Sabatino (1985) consider capacity and competence from a more philosophical level of analysis.

A second level of focus is on the ways that elderly approach their decision making. Beisecker (1988) emphasizes that older persons are less likely to pursue doctors aggressively, and so may operate with less information than would be optimal. Frankl et al. (1989) and Kinsella and Stocking (1989) support that assertion by showing clearly that most elderly (and non-elderly) who may need to make decisions do not discuss those important issues with physicians; the responsibility for this lack of communication appears to lie in both directions. All these authors, however, indicate that the desire of elderly to be involved and informed is strong.

A third focus turns to the kinds of decisions that elderly patients make about health care decisions. It appears clear that older persons are at least as likely or more likely than other patients to prefer <u>not</u> to be given life-sustaining treatment, especially if the prognosis is poor (Diamond et al. for nursing home patients who were capable of decisions, Frankl et al. for terminal and non-terminal inpatients, and Zweibel and Cassel (1989) for outpatients). In several cases, the preferences for care were related to decisions that would be made by surrogates or proxies (someone selected to make the decision about an incompetent person); in most of these cases, the surrogates would make more "overtreatment" choices compared to the elderly themselves (Uhlmann, Pearlman, & Cain, 1988; Zweibel & Cassel, 1989).

If we turn to the role of surrogates, we find that elderly definitely prefer family members to perform that role if needed (High, 1990; Diamond et al., 1989; Tomlinson et al., 1990; Uhlmann et al., 1988). In turn, family members want to be closely involved in decisions (Deimling et al., 1990). Combined with the preference of family members to have more treatment for their elderly relatives than the elderly seem to want (and their belief that their perceptions are accurate), this leads to the need for a much clearer level of communication among family and elderly persons and a very direct emphasis on the role of family members as that of "substituted judgment" rather than an expression of their own wishes or their assumptions about what is best for their family members. Substituted judgment requires that the surrogate correctly identify the preference of the now-incompetent family member, not to express their own personal preference or values (Tomlinson et al., 1990). The same hold true for medical staff, since several of the studies show that physicians have at best a moderate level of knowledge of individual patient preferences and Wettle et al. (1988) indicate that nurses are not very accurate in even predicting how much information older patients know, much less what they desire at a specific level.

Overall, these studies and related work show how far we have yet to go in determining what individual patients want in what is intrinsically a changing situation and in finding the proper mechanisms to insure that patient autonomy about treatment is maintained as much as possible.

RELATED READINGS

Besdine, R. W.(1983). Decisions to withhold treatment from nursing home residents. Journal of the American Geriatrics Society, 31, 602-606.

Davis, A. J.(1989). Clinical nurses' ethical decision making in situations of informed consent. Advances in Nursing Science, 11, 63-69.

DeWolf, M. S.(1989). Ethical decision-making. Seminars in Oncology Nursing, 5, (2), 77-81.

Ruark, J. E. & Raffin, T. A.(1988). Initiating and withdrawing life support: Principles and practices in adult medicine. The New England Journal of Medicine, 318, 25-30.

ANNOTATED BIBLIOGRAPHY

3-1. Beisecker, A.L. (1988). Aging and the desire for information and input in medical decisions: Patient consumerism in medical encounters. Gerontologist, 28, 330-335.

A sample of 106 outpatient rehabilitation patients ranging in age from 17 to over 60 with various ailments were surveyed to measure perceptions of the patient role which might be termed consumerist. The results of the study indicate that as age increased, there was a decreased tendency to believe it was a good idea to suggest alternative treatments and a greater likelihood that a patient desired to put himself completely in the hands of the doctor. Older patients were less likely to challenge a doctor's authority; more likely to place the locus of authority strongly in the hands of the doctor; and overwhelmingly desired information about a wide range of medical areas.
Companions usually accompanied the older patient and the companions made consumerist comments to the physician. Further research should include the effect of this companion on the behavior of the patient and the physician. An important point emerging from this study is despite the fact that elderly patients take on a passive role while interacting with a physician, the desire for information regarding their treatment remains strong.

3-2. Deimling, G.T., Smerglia, V.L., & Barresi, C.M. (1990). Health care professionals and family involvement in care-related decisions concerning older patients. Journal of Aging and Health, 2, 310-325.

The purpose of this research was to examine care-related decisions that are part of the day-to-day caregiving process and to identify the correlates of physician involvement and centrality in the decision-making process. Also addressed was the impact of that involvement on family members' satisfaction with the overall caring process. The data from 244 family caregivers was analyzed showing that 40% of the elders and 53% of the nuclear kin are key decision makers. The results indicate that families prefer to control care-related decisions in the home. Physicians, however, were found to be involved in nearly one fourth of the decision-making processes, but were rarely identified as the most important person involved. Family members caring for older patients with greater levels of impairment, less depressed caregivers and more highly educated caregivers more likely had a physician involved in care-related decisions. Caregivers who included a physician on the decision-making network were on the average significantly more satisfied with the overall caregiving process than those who did not. Positively correlated with physician centrality in decision making was shared living arrangements between elder and caregiver. Elder functioning was negatively correlated with physician centrality in decision making.

Information on the specific nature of decisions involving each member of the network would have enhanced this study. Further research to examine the importance of different individuals (older patient, family member, health care provider) in specific types of decision is warranted.

3-3.   Diamond, E.L., Jernigan, J.A., Moseley, R.A., Messina, V., & McKeown, R.A. (1989). Decision-making ability and advance directive preferences in nursing home patients and proxies. The Gerontologist, 29, 622-626.

To assess decision-making capability and preferences regarding advance directives or living wills, the researchers studied 39 nursing home patients and proxies. Demographic data and functional abilities were obtained from the patient's chart. The interviewer evaluated decisional capacity by utilizing a semistructured interview and then rated the responses in six areas of mental competence. The Mini-Mental State Exam was administered, followed by an assessment of abstract reasoning and judgment. The interviewer then rated decisional capacity as capable, borderline, or incapable. Following the mental status assessment, a structured interview addressed advance directives. The residents were given the opportunity to sign a living will and designate a proxy at the end of the interview. The proxies received an advance directive structured interview similar to the residents.

Residents perceived as decisionally capable were more likely to decline life-prolonging interventions than those perceived incapable. About half of the subjects had given prior thought to terminal-status decisions, but only six recalled signing a declaration. Nineteen of the residents chose to sign the advance directive declaration at the end of the interview. Proxies named included spouses, children, siblings and friends. About half of the proxies had prior discussion with the patient about life-sustaining treatment. Proxies indicated that they were usually very sure of their substituted judgment (70%) and only three proxies indicated a need for the physician to broach the matter.

Obviously, the small sample size is a limitation of the study. The results, however, support the fact that nursing home residents have given prior thought to end of life treatment desires and are willing to provide input into their plan of care.

3-4. Fitten, L.J., Lusky, R., & Hamann, C. (1990). Assessing treatment decision-making capacity in elderly nursing home residents. Journal of the American Geriatrics Society, 38, 1097-1104.

The purpose of this research project was to examine the medical decision-making capacity of a group of aged nursing home residents through the use of pointed clinical vignettes, to explore the relationship between residents' decision-making capacity and assessed mental and physical status and to evaluate the efficacy of grief mental status screening examinations and clinical impressions in identifying those with limited decision-making capacity. A total of 51 subjects, aged 60 or older, completed the study.

Medical decision-making capacity was independently assessed using an instrument that employs vignettes specifically developed for this purpose by the authors. The first vignette related to the use of a hypnotic drug; the second vignette dealt with an invasive diagnostic procedure; and the final vignette addressed the choice of cardiopulmonary resuscitation. Each vignette was read to the participant twice, and any questions about the material were answered. Mental status was measured with two commonly used instruments, Mini-Mental State Exam (MMSE) and Short Portable Mental Status Questionnaire (SPMSQ). Nursing staff rated the participants' level of functional dependence using Katz's Activities of Daily Living and Lawton and Brody's Instrumental Activities of Daily Living. Patient records were also reviewed for sociodemographic information and the primary physician's opinion regarding the patient's ability to give consent for oral surgery, the only assessment of decisional capacity regularly recorded in the charts.

Of the nursing home residents participating, about three quarters were judged by their physicians to be capable of consenting to dental treatment, but only one third achieved a perfect score on the decision-making capacity vignette instrument. Moderately strong and statistically significant levels of association between the residents' decision-making capacity and their performance on cognitive measures were shown by correlational analysis; however, measures of association between functional dependence and decision-making capacity were low and not significant. Judged against the more direct assessment of decision-making capacity developed by the authors, primary physicians' judgment of capacity for consent was 31% to 39% sensitive in identifying impaired decision-making and the MMSE was 53% to 63% sensitive.

The results of this study seem to indicate, at least with this small sample, that measures of direct assessment, rather than indirect assessment, should be utilized in the nursing home population.

3-5. Frankl, D., Oye, R.K., & Bellamy, P.E. (1989). Attitudes of hospitalized patients toward life support: A survey of 200 medical inpatients. <u>American Journal of Medicine</u>, <u>86</u>, 645-648.

Beginning with the basic concept that autonomy of patients concerning treatment is central, Frankl et al. focused on the extent and accuracy of communication of direct information. They presented 200 inpatients at a university hospital with four scenarios, indicating a descending range of likely outcomes of medical intervention, ranging from return to usual activity to persistent vegetative state.

Ninety percent of respondents would desire treatment if it led to a usual level of activity, with reduced levels for other outcomes (30% if dependent, 16% if hopeless, and 6% if in a coma). The researchers divided the subjects by median split into high or low preference for life support and found that females, older persons, and those with terminal diagnoses preferred somewhat less aggressive treatment, although not to extremely large degrees. For example, 66% of those over 65 were in the low treatment choice group, whereas 51% of those under 65 were. Also, amount of discussion and preferred level of discussion with physicians was investigated, showing that only 16% had discussed these issues with their physicians, whereas an additional 47% wished to do so.

This study provides some important information about two facets of health care decision making, illustrating the major difference between desire for communication and actual level of communication and also showing the impact of likely outcome on decisions of patients. Age differences are also interesting. However, the approach to the data was quite weak, especially summing over the scenario situations and the use of median splits rather than using the full range of responses. It is difficult to know whether most respondents want aggressive treatment with some outcomes and none with others or a moderate level of treatment across a range of outcomes or to know whether, for example, most elderly are less oriented to treatment than non-elderly or whether many elderly prefer treatment at least as aggressive as non-elderly but a few were extremely lower on treatment scores than younger persons.

3-6. High, D.M. (1990). Who will make health care decisions for me when I can't? <u>Journal of Aging and Health</u>, <u>2</u>, 291-309.

Comparisons were made between those elderly who have families and those who do not have families regarding the use and interest in advance directives and proxy appointments in this exploratory, qualitative study. Seventy-one elderly men and women were interviewed using a semistructured instrument that encouraged open-ended conversations.

Approximately 50% of each group had talked to someone about what they would want in medical care should they become terminally ill. This number dropped in half for participants without families, however, when asked if they had spoken to anyone about medical care in the event they could not make their own decisions and long-term care would be necessary. Most of the participants had heard of and understood the purpose of a living will; however, only a few people had executed one. Almost all of those without families had used a power of attorney for property and financial management. These power of attorney appointments were not utilized for health care decisions. Elderly persons with relatives consistently expressed preferences for family members to serve as surrogate health care decision makers. This preference for family surrogates exhibited a pattern of hierarchal ordering. Seventy percent of married participants indicated a desire for their spouses, some together with children, as their preferred surrogate. Adult children were next in surrogate preference order, followed by siblings and other family members.

A theme concerning the elderly's preference and expectation to rely informally on family members to make surrogate health care decisions emerges from the data. If the elderly are allowed to voice their preference for informal reliance on family surrogates regarding health care decision making, then patient autonomy remains intact. Elderly people without family members should be encouraged to extend their powers of attorney to include health care decisions.

3-7. Kinsella, T. D., & Stocking, C. B. (1989). Failed communication about life-support therapy: Silent physicians and mute patients. American Journal of Medicine, 86, 643-644.

In an editorial introduction to the issue that includes Frankl et al. (see 3-5), an M. D. and an ethicist discuss the implications of the major findings of that study that possible outcomes are major determinants of choice of treatment or non-treatment and that most physicians and patients do not discuss those options adequately. They point out that significant minorities of patients in the study expressed a lack of desire to have any discussions with physicians about these matters. Thus, Kinsella and Stocking feel that at least some of the blame directed to physicians for not raising life support issues is unwarranted; rather, physicians and patients both should be ready to raise and deal with the issues.

They also point out that a big question continues to be unanswered: are the decisions expressed by patients at one point in time stable across time, or do individuals waver dependent on their own condition and other factors? In regard to that question, they take the position that it is important to narrow the communication gap by working with both physicians and patients and that at the least there should be required periodic reaffirmation of expressed wishes of patients.

3-8. Lo, B. (1990). Assessing decision-making capacity. Law, Medicine & Health Care, 18, 193-201.

In this article, the author discusses the difference between the terms capacity and competence. The latter is a legal category in which there appears to be no clear legal standards for determining whether a person is competent to make medical decisions. This lack of clear standards stems from landmark case rulings usually involving unconscious or severely demented patients with a focus of whether treatment should be given, not whether the patient is competent. Incompetence is usually inferred from a person's overall ability to function in life. The author questions if it would be more appropriate to view incompetence in specific rather than general terms as a person may be capable of performing some tasks adequately, but not others.

The term incapacity is used to refer to assessments by physicians that patients lack the ability to make informed decisions about their health care. A person who is determined to be incapacitated may lose decision-making power in an effort to protect himself or herself from serious harm that may result from those decisions. Physicians have an ethical obligation to use their expertise for the benefit of patients. This obligation to protect conflicts with a physician's obligation to respect the autonomy of persons to make decisions that others might regard as foolish, unwise, or harmful. In assessing decision-making capacity, physicians must balance protecting patients from harm with respecting their autonomy. The author reviews sliding scales suggested for such assessments, philosophers' assessment of a series of abilities to make a decision, the role of mental status testing and psychiatric evaluation. Also mentioned are ways in which health care providers can enhance the decision-making capacity of elderly patients. Case study examples are effectively used to illustrate the concepts the author is trying to stress in this well-written article.

3-9. Sabatino, C.P. (1985). Decision-making mechanisms. Taking Charge of the End of Your Life - Proceedings of a Forum on Living Wills and other Advance Directives (pp. 21-26). Washington, DC: American Bar Association's Commission on Legal Problems of the Elderly and Older Women's League.

The author, on behalf of the American Bar Association's Commission on Legal Problems of the Elderly, presents a broad overview of the larger continuum within which decision-making mechanisms regarding terminal illness exist. The base-line decision-making mechanism is the individual - within the law, a person has the prerogative of making choices based on his own values and beliefs. Only in rare circumstances have the courts authorized treatment against the wishes of a competent patient. These exceptions have generally involved cases where the patient is responsible for a dependent child or where an otherwise healthy person had attempted suicide. Decision-making that departs from the baseline includes power of attorney, trusts, advance directives, proxy consent, quardianship, protective services and ethics committees. The author reviews, in layman's terms, a definition, voluntary or involuntary delegation as well as the legality of each mechanism. This article is a copy of a verbal presentation delivered in Washington, D.C., at a forum on living wills and other advance directives. It is the author's hope that discussions, such as this forum, will spark a significant growth spurt in the understanding of these particular decision making-tools.

3-10. Tomlinson, T., Howe, K., Notman, M., & Rossmiller, D. (1990). An empirical study of proxy consent for elderly persons. The Gerontologist, 30, 54-61.

These researchers stress that substituted judgment has been forwarded as the appropriate approach to having surrogates make health care decisions for older persons. In substituted judgment, the goal of the surrogate is to attempt to make the same decision as the incompetent patient would (in comparison to choosing what the surrogate feels would be best). Yet, little is known about how accurate family members, physicians, and others are in being able to approximate the values of the patient.

In this study, a wide range of 43 community-residing elderly were interviewed on two occasions. In the intake interview they gave basic data about themselves and their support network, and their prediction of whether or not those in the network would make medical decisions for them the same as they would for themselves. In the second interview, they responded to three treatment scenarios (based primarily on level of pre-treatment health status) and indicated their choice of treatment or non-treatment and the reasons for their choices. Meanwhile, those whom they had identified in the initial interview (115 for the 43 subjects) were contacted and asked to indicate either their perception of the elderly person's treatment choices (in a substituted judgment condition) or what they think would be best in such a situation. Treatment choice, a weighted decision choice including level of certainty, and the rating of reasons were compared across elderly and their network. The substituted judgment condition produced significantly less difference between the elderly and their potential proxies than did the "generic" condition. At the same time, frequency of contact, elderly's ratings of the related participants, age, gender, type of relationship, or the elderly's designation of preferred proxy did not result in consistent differences. Family members appeared to be better at substituted judgment, but the difference was not significant.

The authors careful review the methodological flaws and hypothetical nature of the study, but feel that the results lead to several specific conclusions.

A specific charge of substituted judgment given to proxies is much more likely to yield actual accuracy to elderly persons' choices, but the specific individual designated (family member, for example) is more a matter of subjective preference than one that will yield a more accurate judgment. Still, since family members or preferred proxies do at least as well as anyone, the burden of proof should be on those who would disallow their participation, because they are emotionally the most closely related. This carefully done study indicates an important avenue for further research as well as a good guide for how to present health care decision issues to a range of proxies for incompetent patients when there is not a clear living will statement from the patient.

3-11. Uhlmann, R.F., Pearlman, R.A., & Cain, K.C. (1988). Physicians' and spouses' predictions of elderly patients' resuscitation preferences. Journal of Gerontology, 43, M115-121.

To better understand the capacity for substituted judgment under circumstances of mental incapacity, the researchers investigated the understanding of patients' resuscitation preferences by potential surrogate decision makers. Specifically, the ability of primary care physicians and patients' spouses to predict preferences of elderly outpatients for resuscitation from cardiac arrest was examined. Two hundred and fifty-eight patients, aged 65 or more, were recruited through medical practices in community, Veterans Administration (VA) and health maintenance organization (HMO) settings. In addition, 105 physicians and 90 spouses of participating patients were also included. Preferences regarding resuscitation decisions were elicited under four health status scenarios followed by a questionnaire. Respondents were asked to score resuscitation preferences on a 5-point Likert scale.

Although more than three-quarters of physicians and spouses surveyed believed their predictions of patients' preferences were accurate, physicians significantly underestimated patients' resuscitation preferences in the scenarios involving chronic lung disease and stroke, whereas they significantly overestimated them in current health/CPR decision. Spouses overestimated patients' preferences in all decisions. In other words, physicians' most common error in the practice setting would be an irrevocable one of "under-resuscitation" in which patients who wished to be resuscitated would not receive that treatment option. In contrast, the most common response error in predicting patients' preference would be one of "over-resuscitation," in which patients who did not want to be resuscitated would be.

The data, limited to the subsample of patients and physicians, suggest that discussions between surrogate decisionmakers and patients would enhance the accuracy of substituted judgment. Furthermore, the results suggest that the lack of discussions, at least in part, may be due to surrogate decisionmakers' perceptions that they understand patients' preferences. Further research efforts need to address the circumstances under which substituted judgments are accurate as well as the development of methods to improve their accuracy.

3-12. Wettle, T., Levkoff, S., Cwikel, J., & Rosen, A. (1988). Nursing home resident participation in medical decisions: Perceptions and preferences. The Gerontologist, 28, 32-38.

A sample of 198 nursing home residents and their 34 primary nurse caregivers were interviewed regarding perceptions and preferences of resident participation in health care decisions. Primarily, the researchers were interested in the current level of participation of residents in medical care decisions and in the specific decision of whether to attempt resuscitation in the case of arrest, the perceived adequacy of resident involvement and their preferences regarding participation in decisions, and the level of concordance between resident preferences and the perceptions of nurses regarding resident preferences. To obtain their data, the researchers utilized a questionnaire which contained both open-ended and closed questions as well as a case vignette addressing do-not-resuscitate (DNR) decisions. The sample was drawn from nine multi-level long-term care facilities and every effort was made to include residents across a range of cognitive abilities to enhance the generalizability of the findings.

About 40% of the residents reported being told everything about their medical condition, whereas about the same number of respondents reported being told very little or nothing. Almost two-thirds of the respondents reported that they wished they could be involved in DNR decisions. Most residents (92.6%) reported they had not been asked about resuscitation and 72.7% reported that they would not wish to be resuscitated. Concordance between residents' and nurses' perceptions was found to be low. Nurses tended to overestimate the adequacy of information provided by the physician as well as the resident's involvement and desire to be involved in the decision process.

The results of this study indicate the need for improved communication between caregiver and care-recipient in the long-term care setting and the need to recognize that nursing home residents would like to have the opportunity to state their wishes regarding resuscitation.

3-13. Zweibel, N.R. & Cassel, C.K. (1989). Treatment choices at the end of life: A comparison of decisions by older patients and their physician-selected proxies. The Gerontologist, 29, 615-621.

The purpose of this research was to examine the ability of middle-generation family members to serve as proxies for older, decisionally incapacitated patients in a broad array of life-sustaining treatment scenarios. The criteria respondents consider important in making decisions about life-extending treatments and prior experiences of respondents with decision making of this type was also explored. Five brief hypothetical case vignettes dealing with ventilation, resuscitation, chemotherapy, amputation and tube feeding were presented in structured, personal interviews with 55 elderly outpatient/proxy pairs and 52 additional proxies. The proxy was usually a child, niece, or nephew reported to be the most likely to assist the patient with health care needs and who lived within one hour travel time of the outpatient clinic. Spouse proxies were excluded. Therefore, findings cannot be generalized to older persons for whom decisions are made by spouses.

The results indicate that a proportion of pairs in which the patient would want the proxy to make a decision opposite the one the proxy reported he/she would make ranges from 24% for tube feeding and up to 44% and 50% respectively for resuscitation and chemotherapy. Most of the disagreements reflected pairs in which the patient would not want life extension but the proxy would ask for the treatment if left up to him/her. However, in 70% of the disagreements with treatment wishes on the use of resuscitation, the patient would want to be resuscitated, but the proxy would request a do-not-resuscitate order be written. A majority of patients and proxies reported that they had had experiences with a decision similar to those described in the vignettes. Lack of mental acuity and being a burden on family emerged as the two criteria important to all respondents when asked to make decisions about life-extending treatment. Both groups discounted patient age as being important.

A limitation to this study is the questionable strength of a link between projected treatment preferences and those made in the face of actual life-threatening illness. However, this area of concern should not compromise the concordance between patient and proxy choices.

4

DO NOT RESUSCITATE POLICIES IN LONG-TERM CARE FACILITIES

Kristin A. Thomas

INTRODUCTION

Chapter Three introduced a number of major issues concerned with how older persons, their families, and their physicians make decisions about appropriate treatment. The articles cited in this chapter focus more directly on one aspect of treatment decisions-- whether or not to make attempts to resuscitate individuals. The primary type of resuscitation effort is CPR, cardio-pulmonary resuscitation, and many of the items deal with this particular treatment. However, other methods of resuscitation may also be involved.

The most often used vehicle to indicate whether or not resuscitation efforts should be aggressively pursued is the DNR order, or "no code." The existence of such an order indicates that cardiac arrest, for example, will not be responded to even though the non-response will result in death. It is clear that DNR is a specific way to honor living will guidelines or family requests that an individual be allowed to die with dignity (see Chapter 3).

Before considering the main themes and approaches of the presentations cited, it should be noted that the issue of DNR has been given a large push to the forefront of awareness by the OBRA (Omnibus Budget Reconciliation Act) regulations that have recently become effective. OBRA regulations require that specific indications by patients of their wishes concerning use of resuscitation be solicited by health care personnel upon entry to a health care institution and subsequently respected if the occasion arises. The full impact of these regulations is as yet unclear, but while the articles reviewed here were published prior to the regulations, they contain the framework for discussing and implementing the regulations.

One set of readings (Cassel, 1989; Murphy, 1985; Pohlman, 1989, and Tomlinson & Brody, 1988) are primarily focused on ethical, legal, and moral aspects of making decisions about resuscitation. A second, more practically-oriented set (Brunetti et al, 1990; Levinson et al, 1987; Longo et al, 1988; Miller & Cugliari, 1990; Ryden & Miles, 1987; Sharp & Frederick, 1989) focus more directly on policies; most but not all concern long-term care settings. Most of the more conceptual pieces take note of the difficulty of formulating policies, pointing out the conflicting ideas of parties that may be involved in the decision-- physicians, patients, nurses, family. Several articles are reports of empirical investigations of how many instutitions have policies and what those policies cover. The findings about percentages of long-term care institutions that had policies at the time of the research vary quite widely from study to study (from 83% for Brunetti et al, 1990, to fewer than one out of four found by Miles and Ryden, 1985, and Miller and Cugliari, 1990, while Levinson et al, 1987 found about half had policies). The variation is often due to sampling within a specific state; it is clear that some states have been more aggressive in including such policies in the review process than others. Type of facility is sometimes found to have an effect, with larger facilities and teaching facilities more likely to have policies. Meyers et al (1990) took a different analytic approach, by examining the charts of nursing home patients to see the prevalence of DNR orders. They found that over one fourth of the patients had clear orders; increased age and presence of a surrogate decision-maker were correlated with higher percentages of DNR codes.

As with health care decisions more generally, a number of authors who compared the estimates of quality of life, desire for CPR, and attitude toward resuscitation across hospital or nursing home patients, physicians, other health professionals, and family (Lo et al, 1986; Pearlman & Uhlmann, 1988; Stolman et al, 1990) found consistent differences, often in the direction of physicians estimating quality of life in comparison to patients but at the same time being reluctant to discuss DNR. Shelley et al (1987) used hypothetical studies to examine attitudes of nurses and nursing students and found that they would be inclined to give less aggressive treatment to older persons, regardless of whether or not there were specific DNR orders, and those who had explicit DNR orders.

Taffet, Teasdale, and Luchi (1988) directly examined the effectiveness of resuscitation efforts in a Veterans Administration population and found that older patients were able to be resuscitated but had a lower prognosis of being discharged alive.

Many of the readings make an additional point about how nurses, in particular, are often caught in the middle. They often must provide care to a patient who has little hope of recovery if there is not a DNR order or stand by while a patient with a DNR order dies. They may also bear the heat of family members whose goals conflict with physicians, who are the only ones able to write the orders. Cassel (1989), Dufault (1985), Fowler (1989), Murphy (1985), Pohlman (1989), and Sharp and Frederick (1989) all give considerable attention to the difficult role of nurses in the DNR process.

Given the changing nature of life and death in our society, the changing policy and regulatory arena, the interplay of decision-making and competence in long-term care populations, and the seemingly intrinsically conflicting goals of physicians, family, policymakers, and a variety of health care providers, it is clearly critical to continue to examine and evaluate the factors that lead to and the effects of DNR orders. It is also likely that nurses will continue to be those most caught in the middle when conflicts arise.

RELATED READINGS

American Nurses' Association. (1982). Nursing Practice in the Care of the Dying. Kansas City, MO: Author.

American Nurses' Association. (1985). Code for Nurses with Interpretive Statements. Kansas City, MO: Author.

American Nurses' Association, Committee on Ethics. (1988). Guidelines on Withdrawing or Withholding Food or Fluid. Kansas City, MO: Author.

Brown, N.K. & Thompson, D.J. (1979). Nontreatment of fever in extended-care facilities. The New England Journal of Medicine, 1246-1250.

Emanuel, L.L. (1989). Does the DNR order need life-sustaining intervention? Time for comprehensive advance directives. American Journal of Medicine, 86, 86-87.

Emanuel, L.L. & Emanuel, E.J. (1989). The medical directive. JAMA, 261, 3288-3293.

Fader, A.M., Gambert, S.R., Nash, M., Gupta, K.L., & Escher, J. (1989). Implementing a "do-not-resuscitate" (DNR) policy in a nursing home. Journal of the American Geriatrics Society, 37, 544-548.

Knox, L.S. (1989). Ethical issues in nutritional support nursing. Nursing Clinics of North America, 24, 427-436.

President's Commission for the Study of Ethical Problems in Medicine and Biomedical and Behavioral Research. (1983). Deciding to forego life-sustaining treatment: A report on the ethical, medical, and legal issues in treatment decisions. Washington, DC: U.S. Government Printing Office.

Stenberg, M.J. (1988). "The responsible powerless": Nurses and decisions about resuscitation. Journal of Cardiovascular Nursing, 3, 47-56.

U.S. Congress, Office of Technology Assessment (1987). Life-sustaining technologies and the elderly. OTA-BA 306. Washington, DC: U.S. Government Printing Office, July.

ANNOTATED BIBLIOGRAPHY

4-1. Brunetti, L.L., Weiss, M.J., Studenski, S.A., & Clipp, E.C. (1990). Cardiopulmonary resuscitation policies and practices. Archives of Internal Medicine, 150, 121-126.

In this study, 236 state-registered long-term care facilities in North Carolina were surveyed to determine the prevalence of written cardiopulmonary resuscitation policies. Over eighty-eight percent of the facilities responded to the questionnaire revealing that 83% of the respondents had written policies. A content analysis was also performed on the 86 copies of policies that had been provided by the nursing homes. The written policies were systematically compared with 10 model criteria. It was found that policy content varied substantially. Provisions for authorization, informed consent, documentation, competency, review, and applicability of do not resuscitate orders were contained in over half of the policies. Less than half, however, contained criteria for autonomy, treatment alternatives, dignity and quality of care, as well as patient identification. Nursing facilities that had written policies were newer, larger, and for-profit; had a greater proportion of skilled nursing care beds; and were more likely to have both Medicare and Medicaid certification.

The researchers accomplished the goals they set out to do in this descriptive study. In this study, the researchers enjoyed a high return rate on their questionnaires. Perhaps this phenomenon was due to the fact that a separate letter had been mailed to the administrators of the facilities from the North Carolina Health Care Facilities Association encouraging participation in the study. The authors used a Model Policy Criteria to systematically compare the written policies. This model centered around ethical and legal principles and procedural provisions. Inclusion of these 10 policy criteria in a comprehensive cardiopulmonary resuscitation policy would represent an important step toward enhancing the quality of decision making by nursing home residents. The variations represented in these policies place nursing home residents at risk of having important personal rights limited or ignored. It will be of interest to note if the new Medicare reimbursement regulations effective October 1, 1990, with a focus on allowing nursing home residents to make choices and improvements on quality of life, will have any bearing on the results of future studies on this topic.

4-2. Cassel, C.K. (1989). Care of the dying: The limits of law, the limits of ethics. Law, Medicine & Health Care, 17, 232-233.

Dr. Cassel provides commentary on the limits of law and ethics in health care. She first gives a brief history of the problems of death and dying stemming from the early 1970's. The advent of growth in medical technology in the decade of the 1960's, the author notes, amplified the denial of death in American hospitals and among medical professionals themselves. As a result, grassroots efforts called for more humane treatment and the right to die with dignity. Statutory changes began with California's Natural Death Act in 1976. Soon after the first American hospices emerged and Karen Ann Quinlan's parents successfully appealed to the courts to allow her ventilator to be discontinued.

Now, over two decades after the first concerns were raised, hospice care, living wills, durable powers of attorney, and advance directives have been utilized and improved on throughout the United States. Cassel points out that many fear that the pendulum has swung too far and that cost-containment pressures will allow patients to die prematurely for reasons of convenience or economy rather than caring or compassion. He believes that the inability to care fully for the dying in our society has deep social, cultural, and, perhaps, religious roots and cannot be easily dealt with by the structural provisions of the law or the rational analysis of biomedical ethics. Cassel also directs her concerns to the medical profession, which she feels must begin to view death as a part of life and see its special role in the dying process. The author warns that physicians can never expect complete legal immunity or to have all of the answers laid out by hospital policies, state law, or specialty and professional societies. Physicians must have the courage to do this difficult task and not to expect that the difficult task will ever become easy.

Overall, this article provides a reasoned overview of the issues involved in legal and ethical aspects of the timing of death in a technological society.

4-3. Dufault, K. (1985). What is nurses role when adults forego treatment? In American Nurses' Association Committee on Ethics (Eds.), Ethical Dilemmas Confronting Nurses, 7-10. Kansas City, MO: American Nurses' Association.

As a member of the American Nurses' Association Committee on Ethics, the author recognizes the increasing number of issues surrounding the care of adult patients and decisions related to life-sustaining treatment. These complex issues are associated with advances in technology that provide the capability for postponing death even when there is no reasonable expectation of improving well-being. The author briefly addresses the issues of underlying conflicting moral values of participants in the decision-making process, including informed consent and competency, and the controversy that exists over what constitutes life-sustaining treatment in ethical, legal and moral arenas.

The nurse's role has been identified to include the responsibility to be informed about and to participate in decision-making related to institutional policies that deal with life-sustaining treatment. This nursing responsibility requires knowledge of the role and function of the institutional ethics committee as well. Nurses act to enhance the persons' ability to make decisions on their own behalf - with the nurse providing information on current condition, treatment options available and providing assistance in weighing the benefits or burdens of treatment. The nurse must also help identify and locate appropriate others to make decisions when the person is not able to make an informed choice. Once the decision has been made to forgo life-sustaining treatment, nursing care is then focused on the prevention alleviation of suffering, commonly accompanying the dying process. The author concludes it will be the nursing care the individual receives that will determine to a great degree how this finale of human experience is lived and the peace and dignity with which death is approached.

4-4. Fowler, M.D.M. (1989). Slow code, partial code, limited code. <u>Heart & Lung</u>, <u>18</u>, 533-534.

Fowler provides commentary on ethical dilemmas in critical care. Cardiopulmonary resuscitation (CPR) refers to measures that are highly intrusive, and some are violent in nature. The author points out a number of factors that weigh in one's determination that CPR in the light of the patient's condition, the violence of the procedure and the burden of its sequelae to the patient, and the patient's wishes or the family's desires to do what would be in the best interest of the patient. These factors, the author believes, should result in a clearly defined plan for CPR or DNR. It should, but it often does not. Instead, the author notes, our health care system is left with vagueness and confusion related to resuscitation orders or lack of them.

The vagueness ensues because of relationships formed between health-care workers and long-term patients and the resulting inability to "let go," in which patient death is seen as a failure, as well as the threat litigation. As a result, the nursing care unit is plagued with "slow code," "partial code" and "limited code" orders that can be looked as a dishonest effort that needs to be justified by reasons stronger than merely the providers' discomfort in discussing DNR decisions. The author makes the important point that health care providers need to look at more effective ways of coping with family grief. It is also important to point out that health care delivery systems must also be attentive to the grieving needs of health care workers as well.

4-5. Gleeson, K. & Wise, S. (1990). The do-not-resuscitate order. Archives of Internal Medicine, 150, 1057-1060.

The charts of 274 consecutive deaths in a Pennsylvania Medical Center were reviewed to examine the approach of physicians, patients, and families in making the decision to invoke the "do-not-resuscitate" (DNR) order. Of the 274 patients who had died, 62% had do-not-resuscitate orders. Half of those with DNR orders were judged to be fully mentally competent on admission to the hospital; 51% of the fully mentally competent patients were included in the decision to withhold resuscitative efforts. In the remainder, the family was usually involved in efforts. In the remainder, the family was usually involved in the decision without input from the patient. Only 6 patients were admitted to the hospital with a pre-existing DNR order. Presence of terminal disease was the principal reason cited for a DNR order (52%), followed by an unacceptable quality of life (33%). Nursing activities were quantified for the 24 hours preceding and the 24 hours following the DNR order. Comparing these two periods, whether on a general ward or an intensive care unit, no difference in nursing activity was found.

This study extends observations from previous studies. The DNR order has become routine before anticipated in hospital death. The patient is frequently not involved in this decision and this commonly seems to be a result of impaired mental status. The findings reflect the continued disinclination of physicians to broach this issue with their chronically ill patients before their hospital admission. The percentage of patients involved in the DNR decision in this study exceeds that of previous reports.

There are several limitations in this study as noted by the authors. Assessment of mental status was made at admission and not when the DNR order was actually written. The possibility of a mentally competent individual's status deteriorating along with one's physical condition often exists. The results of the study depend critically on the accuracy of documentation on the record. As a result, the researchers relied heavily on standardized admission forms. The researchers also note that their measure of nursing activity is clearly flawed as it is possible for the check marks on the nurses' activity sheet inaccurately reflect actual nursing activity. This study only analyzes the quantitative aspects related to a DNR order and does not describe the qualitative factors such as spiritual well-being, counseling and meaning of death to those involved.

4-6. Levinson, W., Shepard, M.A., Dunn, P.M., & Parker, D.F. (1987). Cardiopulmonary resuscitation in long term care facilities: A survey of do-not-resuscitate orders in nursing homes. Journal of the American Geriatrics Society, 35, 1059-1062.

The state of Oregon's total population of long-term care facilities was surveyed. The purpose of the survey was to identify how nursing homes currently manage issues related to cardiopulmonary resuscitation (CPR). Of the 76 facilities, it was found that 41% had a DNR policy and of those without such a policy, 70% felt that some type of protocol was needed. Forty-three percent of the respondents reported that discussions of limited treatment and resuscitation included residents and their families. This discussion was most likely presented by the registered nurse responsible for care or by the attending physician. Most of the facilities recorded the DNR order by the attending physician as a written order and the DNR designation was most commonly displayed inside or on the front of the resident's chart. No significant difference in having a policy or in discussing and recording no-CPR orders was found between nonprofit and proprietary facilities, between small (less than 100 beds) and large (more than 100 beds) facilities, or between facilities better prepared for resuscitation (those that required basic life support training for staff members or those that had an emergency cart available). Most facilities had oxygen and suction equipment: approximately one half had the capability to give intravenous medications or to use hand-held ventilation equipment. CPR certification was reported by the majority as a requirement for the nursing staff, however, only one half said they had a recertification policy.

Policies surrounding CPR issues are important. The capability of a nursing home to perform CPR and other life-saving treatment is crucial. This study points out that long-term care delivery also needs to work on their ability to provide life-saving treatment for those residents requesting these services. This may help to improve the quality of resident care and lessen potential conflicts for those involved.

4-7. Lo, B., McLeod, G. A., & Saika, G. (1986). Patient attitudes to discussing life-sustaining treatment. Archives of Internal Medicine, 146, 1613-1615.

One hundred and fifty-two ambulatory patients in a university-based general medical practice filled out questionnaires on advance directives, surrogate decision making and the care desired if he or she should become severely demented. The patients were placed into three study groups: 1 included 28 patients under 65 years with cancer, angina pectoris, congestive heart failure, chronic obstructive lung disease, stroke, cirrhosis, or chronic renal failure; group 2 included 69 patients, 65 years or older, with these diagnoses; and group

3 included 55 patients with mental impairment were excluded from the study.

Sixty-six percent of the respondents had thought quite a lot or a moderate amount about when they would want to make decisions, and 13% preferred their physicians, however, only 9% had spoken with their physician about surrogate decision makers. Age was the only variable significantly related to thoughts of surrogate decision makers with those patients over 65 thinking about this topic more often than younger patients. Sixty-two percent had thought quite a lot or a moderate amount what treatment they would want if they suffered from confusion, severe memory loss and inability to take care of themselves with no chance of recovery. A majority of these respondents would refuse intensive treatment, CPR, feeding tubes and half would refuse antibiotics and hospitalization for pneumonia. About half of these respondents had discussed their treatment desires with relatives. Age was the only variable found to be significantly related to thoughts of surrogate decision making and the refusal of treatment. Those over 65 thought about the subject more and declined life-saving treatment at a higher rate. Most respondents indicated a sense of control when discussing life-sustaining treatment. Over half wanted their physician to bring up the matter.

The results of this study may not be reflective of other clinical settings. Patients were only asked about preferences for care if they became severely demented and their preferences may be different in other clinical situations. It is interesting to note that such a high number of ambulatory patients have thought about life sustaining treatment choices. One could speculate about those who are immobile or institutionalized may have given even more thought to end-of-life treatment choices.

The results of a study such as this may show different results if the respondents were acutely ill. Yet, even with these limitations, this careful study shows the depth of interest in and personal decisions about end-of-life treatment choices.

4-8. Longo, D.R., Burmeister, R., & Warren, M. (1988). "Do not resuscitate": Policy and practice in the long-term care setting. Journal of Long-Term Care Administration, Spring, 5-11.

This study surveyed 585 randomly selected long-term care facilities from around the nation about protocols for DNR orders. It was reported that 50.7% had no such policy and of those having policies, only 20% had formal written documents. The long-term care providers with these formal DNR Policies were more likely to include in their policies the withholding of treatment. The areas most frequently addressed through a formal DNR policy in the long-term setting included documentation of the order, specifics about who writes such an order and discussions about DNR need with the resident, family, or guardian. Only 3.7% of the facilities utilized ethics committees. Of the problems found relating to the implementation of DNR policies, the need for staff continuing education on DNR issues was the most frequent problem encountered followed by problems in defining the relationship of DNR to other treatments and legal issues.

The long-term care institutions included in this study are one type of setting in what is a larger study of all health care delivery systems - acute, psychiatric, long-term and hospice care. It is interesting to note that long-term care settings rank second to last (followed by psychiatric facilities) in the extent to which health care institutions have formulated DNR policies.

4-9. Meyers, R.M., Lurie, N., Breitenburger, R.B., & Waring, C.J. (1990). Do-not-resuscitate orders in an extended-care study group. Journal of the American Geriatrics Society, 38, 1011-1015.

The charts of 911 nursing home patients were reviewed in Minnesota to determine the prevalence of do-not-resuscitate (DNR) orders. Data on demographic characteristics, availability of a surrogate decisionmaker as well as participation of a surrogate decision-maker in the decision were collected by the researchers. In all, 27% of the patients had DNR orders; 90% had potentially available surrogate decisionmakers. For 31% of the patients with DNR orders, however, there was no documentation of patient or surrogate participation in the DNR decision. The female sex, increased age, level of care (skilled versus intermediate), presence of a potential surrogate decisionmaker, and increasing length os time since nursing home admission were identified by univariate analysis as factors associated with presence of DNR orders. Independently associated with the presence of DNR status, using a logistic regression model, was increased age, increased length of time since nursing home admission, skilled versus intermediate level of care, and presence of a surrogate decision-maker.

The study was performed in an inpatient extended care program affiliated with a moderately-sized teaching hospital. The medical center uses a standardized form on which the physician records DNR status. DNR orders that originate in the hospital are transferred to the nursing home status forms. The authors, however, did not indicate whether or not the medical center, or any part of it, incorporates a DNR policy which should act as a guide for physicians with issues of informed consent, autonomy, competency and dignity of residents. The researchers did not investigate decision-making capacity and had to rely on the accuracy of documentation. The study adds to the limited knowledge on this topic and provides grounds for further research: to determine if the factors identified that are significantly related to DNR status are used by physicians when advising families about limited treatment plans.

4-10. Miles, S.H. & Ryden, M.B. (1985). Limited treatment policies in long-term care facilities. Journal of the American Geriatrics Society, 33, 707-711.

In this descriptive study, it was found that 67% of long-term care facilities in a random sample of 143 facilities accepted DNR orders when written for a resident and 73% accepted care plans which limited treatment, most limiting emergency care and allowing death to occur. The alleviation of physical discomfort, anxiety, and social isolation were advocated by the protocols. Of those facilities studied only 16.3% had administrative protocols in place, most of them in utilization for two years or less. It was discovered that facilities delivering skilled care, those which had ethics committees, those operated by a church, and teaching facilities were twice as likely to have limited treatment protocols than other facilities. Few facilities advocated routing discussion of limited treatment protocols with the resident and only two facilities performed this discussion upon admission. Only 25% of those responding to the survey described a primary role for the residents in these decisions.

The researchers set out to determine the prevalence and design of administrative protocols for limited plans in Minnesota nursing homes to understand how facilities perceive such decisions and to identify problem areas in policy design. Because of limited information available, a short questionnaire is a good choice for obtaining descriptive data on this topic. The researchers also were able to analyze a majority of the policies - a process that adds a great deal of information to the study, allowing the researchers to meet their goals.

4-11. Miller, J. & Cugliari, A.M. (1990). Withdrawing and withholding treatment: Policies in long-term care facilities. The Gerontologist, 30, 462-468.

The authors, as members of the New York State Task Force on Life and Law, conducted a survey of nursing homes in 1986 and 1988. The survey examined the existence of policies on decisions about life-sustaining treatment, the process to determine which residents have decision-making capacity, the prevalence of ethics committees or vehicles to resolve disputes, and policies on advance directives such as living wills and durable powers of attorney. The responses of the 1986 and 1988 surveys were then compared to show an increase in the number of facilities that have established explicit policies and institutional vehicles to have established explicit policies and institutional vehicles to address the dilemmas associated with decisions to withdraw or withhold life-sustaining treatment.

In 1986, only 19% of those nursing homes surveyed had policies on withholding or withdrawing treatment, however, 24% said that a policy "in progress." In 1988, the number of homes with a life-sustaining treatment policy had risen to 26% and only 9% indicated that the policies were "in progress." CPR was the treatment most commonly addressed by facility policies, followed by artificial respiration and antibiotics in 1986. The majority of the facilities responding in 1988 indicated that facility policies covered artificial nutrition, hydration and respiration, while 22% addressed the use of antibiotics. The 1988 survey also sought additional information about institutional policies - almost all policies were written and most covered decisions to transfer residents to other facilities for treatment.

The 1986 survey also covered decision-making capacity. On the average, facilities who responded estimated that 26% of the residents had full capacity, 26% had partial capacity and 47% had no capacity. Skilled nursing facilities reported lower capacity levels among residents. This area of the questionnaire was not repeated because the data was consistent with national studies and it was not believed the estimate would change over time. It was not mentioned if there was a tool utilized in determining mental capacity or who determined capacity. These numbers may be inaccurate if the person estimating is untrained in determining capacity or if the person has little contact with the residents. In both years, facilities reported that the attending physician is involved in virtually all cases for decisions regarding life- sustaining treatment for residents who lack capacity. The researchers also found that the number of facilities honoring advance directives such as living wills or durable powers of attorney, increased substantially over the 2-year period even though neither form of advance directive had been formally recognized in New York statutes. The results of both surveys indicated that facilities with ethics committees were more likely to have established institutional policies for the withholding and withdrawal of life-sustaining treatments than were facilities without committees.

Proprietary facilities were underrepresented in both years - the impact of this underrepresentation on the results of study is unclear based on the results of other nursing home surveys performed around the country. The results can only project the general direction that New York State nursing homes are moving. A true longitudinal study could not be performed due to the anonymity of the respondents. Though the results of the study show an increase on the reliance of life-sustaining treatment policies by nursing homes, only a relatively small percentage of facilities in both 1986 and 1988 had policies on this issue.

4-12. Murphy, C.P. (1985). Taking charge of the end of your life. Proceedings of a Forum on Living Wills and other Advance Directives (pp. 44-48). Washington, DC: American Bar Association's Commission on Legal Problems of the Elderly & Older Women's League.

This article was a presentation the author delivered at a Forum on Living Wills and other Advance Directives on behalf of the American Nurses'

Association (ANA) Committee on Ethics. The author acknowledges that many members of the nursing profession are in a position to observe, assess and seriously affect the quality of life of their patients. As a direct caregiver, the nurse may have the traditional moral duty to preserve life when there is a reasonable hope of doing so. Yet, at the same time, the nurse is morally obligated to foster patient self-determination by respecting the patient's choice to reject treatment that may prolong or enhance the quality of his or her life. The ANA code of ethics serves as a contract between society and the profession by explicitly setting forth the values and ethical principles which guide the actions of practicing professionals. The code acts as a framework from which nurses can make ethical decisions and be held accountable to nursing colleagues and the public for their actions. Conflict also arises for nurses when they perceive that aggressive medical treatment is being provided to patients who have no real hope of recovery for a meaningful existence in the long run. This dilemma often occurs when physicians place emphasis on pathological cellular functioning while nurses may be focusing on a more holistic approach on quality of life issues.

The author also reviews three nonpublished Master's Studies performed at Boston College related to factors that influence nurses' decision-making about resuscitation. The patient's prior and present wishes; prognosis of survival; the patient's current degree of pain or suffering; likelihood of recovery to an acceptable quality of life; certainty of the patient's competence in order to make an informed decision and written documentation of do-not-resuscitate orders were critical factors in all three studies.

4-13. Pearlman, R.A. & Uhlmann, R.F. (1988). Quality of life in chronic diseases: perceptions of elderly patients. Journal of Gerontology, 43, M25-30.

In order to better characterize a patient's quality of life, 126 elderly outpatients with five common chronic diseases and their physicians were interviewed. Specifically, the researchers studied patient quality of life assessments, and the attributes and events that affect quality of life so that physicians could better understand it. The researchers where also interested in whether outpatients assessed their quality of life to be different across common chronic diseases, and if so, why. Criteria to participate in the study included 1) age equal or greater than 65 years; 2) presence of at least one chronic disease; 3) at least one visit to their physician in the last 6 months, and two visits in the last year; 4) not demented; and 5) not terminally ill.

Physicians consistently gave lower global ratings of patient quality of life than patients did across all chronic diseases and at all health care settings. Weak associations between physician and patient rating of patient quality of life provides further evidence of limited physician understanding of patient quality of life. Differences in patient ratings of quality of life across chronic diseases were not statistically significant. Patients with cancer and ischemic heart disease tended to view their quality of life slightly worse than did diabetes and arthritis patients. Physicians, however considered quality of life to be significantly worse in patients with cancer and ischemic heart disease. Responding to open-ended questions, patients emphasized medical care, health-related problems and interpersonal relationships as factors affecting quality of life included health, financial concerns, psychological distress (depression and anxiety) and relationships.

The small sample size of this study is a limitation and, therefore, may not be representative of elderly outpatients. This study, however, points out the importance of involving the elderly person in health care decisions, especially ones related to quality of life.

4-14. Pohlman, K.J. (1989). Legal issues in nursing. DNR? CPR? Focus on Critical Care, 16, 224-225.

This article reviews the current law regarding resuscitation and refusal or withdrawal of treatment. The author begins by addressing two questions commonly asked by a nurse: are DNR decisions legal? and (2) must CPR always be initiated? It is recommended that the nurse must first become familiar with the applicable state laws as well as the employer's policies. Beyond that, the answers are based on an understanding of the legal background concerning patient rights.

Most states recognize a common-law right to self-determination and have adopted various approaches that allow an incompetent patient to refuse treatment, often through a surrogate decision maker. Living wills and durable powers of attorney are also recognized in most jurisdictions. The author stated that these legal developments all support the exercise of an individual's right to refuse treatment, including life-saving treatment. A DNR order is considered to be legal if it is thought to be a proper medical treatment option, if it is based on informed consent of the resident, and if it is written or co-signed by the physician in compliance with the appropriate state law. If a nurse discovers a patient unresponsive and no legal DNR decision exists, policy usually requires the initiation of CPR, whether or not it was a witnessed emergency.

This article is brief; however, it provides a concise overview of the legal aspects of DNR orders and fully addresses the two life-sustaining treatment questions commonly asked by caregivers.

4-15. Ryden, M.B. & Miles, S.H. (1987). Limiting treatment in long-term care facilities: The need for policies or guidelines. The Journal of Long Term

Care Administration, Spring, 23-26.

This very brief article discusses the need for guidelines or policies for limiting treatment in long-term care facilities and proposes an outline for the content of such policies or guidelines. The authors base the need for limited treatment policies on the fact that nearly one-fourth of all deaths of persons over 65 occur in nursing homes. Fear of litigation and uncertainty over policy construction, however, have made long-term care administrators cautious in the area of policy development. The authors review needed content of protocols, care plan construction and documentation procedures. The authors base their recommendations for policy development on their survey findings (Miles & Ryden, 1985) regarding DNR policies.

4-16. Sharp, J.Q. & Frederick, B.J. (1989). Developing do not resuscitate policies. Journal of Nursing Administration, 19, 25-29.

The authors, as part of a Nursing Service Task Force, prepared materials for an interdisciplinary medical center do-not-resuscitate (DNR) policy review. Entering into DNR policy development with the sole objective of meeting the recent Joint Commission for the Accreditation Health Care Organizations (JCAHO) standards is, in the author's opinion, short-sighted. Instead, they feel the time spent in policy development should lay the groundwork for understanding the complex treatment and nontreatment issues confronting the health care team. The authors believe the goal of the DNR policy should be to build systems that support staff in the delivery of quality patient care and anticipate the difficult ethical and legal situations of the future.

The authors review the historical perspective of CPR, the JCAHO standards, committee composition for developing the policy, steps for policy development, national trends and future issues related to DNR policies. Woven throughout this overview is the communication to reduce ethical and legal dilemmas. The authors urge nurse administrators to take a leadership role in developing a DNR policy.

4-17. Shelley, S.I., Zahorchak, R.M., & Gambrill, C.D.S. (1987). Aggressiveness of nursing care for older patients and those with do-not-resuscitate orders. Nursing Research, 36, 157-162.

The following hypotheses were tested: 1) DNR orders reduce aggressiveness of nursing care, 2) increased age reduces aggressiveness of nursing care, and 3) patient age and DNR orders interact to affect aggressiveness of nursing care. Two independent variables, DNR orders and age, were manipulated using four vignettes which were randomly assigned to 95 staff nurses in a metropolitan hospital. Two replications with 183 nursing students and 86 intensive care nurses followed. Aggressiveness of care was measured by a 13-item 6-point Likert scale following each vignette which described a specific patient identically except for two variations. Half described the patient as 72 years old, the other half as 28 years. Within each of the two age versions, half described the patient as having DNR orders and the other half did not. Results showed that both increased age and DNR orders significantly reduced aggressiveness of nursing care attitudes in all three studies. A significant interaction between patient age and DNR orders was found. DNR orders resulted in less agreement with aggressive care for the older patient but not the younger among nursing students. The authors attribute this finding to the possible highest level of idealism among students which changes when the realities of daily clinical practice are encountered. Although DNR orders and advanced age resulted in attitudes toward less aggressive care, this level of care remained in the moderately aggressive range indicating that there is no basis relating DNR orders with a poor level of care.

A major limitation to the research technique used in this study is the possible discrepancy between the simulated care behaviors on questionnaires and actual behaviors in a real clinical setting.

4-18.   Stolman, C.J., Gregory, J.J., Dunn, D., & Levine, J.L. (1990). Evaluation of patient, physician, nurse, and family attitudes toward do not resuscitate orders. <u>Archives of Internal Medicine, 150</u>, 653-658.

Attitudes toward resuscitation were investigated by systematically interviewing 97 competent patients classified as "do not resuscitate," 60 physicians, 80 family members and 84 nurses. In addition, 58 family members of incompetent "do not resuscitate" patients were interviewed. The patients interviewed were generally elderly widows with a diagnosis of malignancy. A majority of the patients interviewed preferred that their medical decision making be shared with the physician and/or family members. Only 38 patients could correctly define a "living will," however, after hearing the definition, 59 patients thought it was a good idea to ask noncritically ill patients at the time of admission to a hospital if they had a living will. Fifty-six patients said they had discussed resuscitation with their physicians, whereas, 44 physicians said they had discussed this issue with the patient. Thirty percent of the physicians felt uncomfortable discussing resuscitation with the patients. Over half of the patients (67%) wanted involvement in resuscitation decisions. Forty-nine family members of incompetent patients said they had spoken to their relatives' physicians about resuscitation. A higher percentage of family members of competent patients said they knew their relatives' wishes for resuscitation than did family members of incompetent patients.

The results of this study indicate that physicians and patients have different perceptions of having discussed resuscitation. This discrepancy derives from confounding factors in both physician and patient perception. The patient may become anxious and forgetful when discussing this sensitive topic and the physician may feel guilty over being unable to "save" the patient, for example. The patients interviewed were judged to be competent at the time of interview. For many patients, competency may fluctuate during the course of hospitalization and this may have also influenced physicians' decision to discuss resuscitation. Nurses in this study were consistently found not to be involved in the DNR discussion, possibly due to the nursing shortage, with nurses caring for a greater number of patients and spending less time with each patient ad family than formerly. Alternatively, nurses noninvolvement may be due to political issues which may limit nurses' willingness or ability to get involved in DNR discussion.

The limitations of this study include a small sample size from one community hospital. The data may not be representative of other hospitals and locations. Analyzing a sensitive and complex issue like resuscitation with a simple response format may sacrifice important qualitative data that should be explored.

4-19. Taffet, G.E., Teasdale, T.A., & Luchi, R.J. (1988). In-hospital cardiopulmonary resuscitation. Journal of the American Medical Association, 260, 2069-2072.

Cardiopulmonary resuscitation (CPR) efforts were reviewed retrospectively at a Veterans Administration Medical Center to evaluate the observation that few geriatric patients were discharged alive after they underwent CPR. A total of 399 CPR efforts were made for 329 patients during the study period; a majority of the patients were men. Resuscitative efforts were performed on patients ranging from 25 to 93 years, with a mean age of 62.6 years. It was found that resuscitative efforts for witnessed arrests in which CPR was immediately initiated were more frequently successful than for unwitnessed arrests. The highest percentage of successful resuscitations occurred in the intensive care units; however, the highest percentage who lived to discharge were resuscitated in the emergency department. The presence of sepsis, cancer, increased age, increased number of medication doses administered, and absence of witnesses were shown by multivariate analysis to be "predictive" of poor outcomes. In patients over the age of 70 who had arrests, 24 CPR efforts were successful and 22 patients were alive after 24 hours. None, however, lived to discharge. The authors state the results of their study strongly suggest that older, hospitalized, male patients undergoing a cardiac arrest in a Veterans Hospital, though they survive the CPR effort with the same frequency as younger patients, have a greatly diminished likelihood of being discharged alive.

The primary source of data used for this study was a nursing critique sheet completed by the nurse in attendance shortly after each arrest. The authors also reviewed the hospital chart and the physician's arrest sheet to augment and confirm each nursing critique sheet. The results of this study depend on the accuracy of documentation which may be influenced by the intensity and emotions of an arrest.

4-20. Tomlinson, T. & Brody, H. (1988). Ethics and communication in do-not-resuscitate orders. The New England Journal of Medicine, 318, 43-46.

Tomlinson and Brody offer three distinct rationales for DNR orders: (a) CPR would be of no medical benefit to the patient - a judgement based solely on the physician's clinical expertise and experience, (b) the patient would suffer a poor quality of life after CPR, and (c) the patient suffers from a poor quality of life before CPR. The authors present these rationales in hopes to clear some of the difficulties often associated with do-not-resuscitate orders. The difficulties include physicians' ambivalence about who should be consulted before a DNR order is written, the frustration of interns and nurses who are asked to continue complicated or invasive treatments on a patient for whom a DNR order has been written, and health-care administrators' uncertainty and confusion over what their DNR policies should be.

The rationales are valuable especially when one examines the contrasts underlying them. The first important difference concerns the relevance of the patient's or appropriate other's values to the justification for the DNR decision. The authors point out that the physician's values may well differ from those of the patient or appropriate other, and since the patient has both a legal and a moral right to accept or refuse treatment in accordance with his or her values, the values used to make the quality of life determinations are properly the patient's. When the rationale is purely a matter of expert judgement, the physician has the right to make the decision.

The other important area of contrast among the three rationales concerns their specificity to the event of an arrest and subsequent resuscitation, and the generalizations they allow about the appropriateness of treatment alternatives besides CPR. A DNR order based on "no medical benefit" and "poor quality of life after CPR" limit the scope of their judgements to CPR. Futility of CPR in these cases does not imply futility for other life-prolonging treatments. On the other hand, a DNR order based on "poor quality of life before CPR" involves a judgement that death would be preferable to continued survival, because of the burdens related to disease or life-prolonging treatment.

5

RITUALS RELATED TO DEATH, DYING AND SERIOUS INFIRMITY: A NURSING BIBLIOGRAPHY

Robert D. Woodcock

INTRODUCTION

This bibliography describes nursing literature which will be helpful to researchers investigating rituals related to serious illness and death. Although some people think of nurses and nursing care exclusively in terms of the medical treatments that nurses administer, the scope of nursing goes well beyond the curing of diseases. Nursing practice includes interventions which focus on a whole range of possible human responses to the health problems which people encounter in life. These responses can be physiological (e.g. edema), emotional (e.g. anxiety), spiritual (e.g. doubting one's faith), or social (e.g. isolation, violence, or changes in the pattern of family life). When a patient experiences such responses to his or her own health problems, they are often called nursing diagnoses. But the person with a health problem is not the only one who might respond to it with some emotional, spiritual, social, or even physiological change. The patient's family and friends, other patients, health care professionals, and others who know or encounter the person with the health problem may also respond with such a change. Some of these changes may be associated with behaviors that become rituals. These behaviors are the focus of this chapter.

Due to the wide variety of disciplines engaged in the study of ritual, no consensus has emerged among scholars concerning the proper definition of the word. As a general guide in selecting the items to be included in this bibliography, the following definition was utilized: Ritual is a prescribed procedure arising out of human interaction and involving a pattern of behavior which tends to occur over and over again in similar form. This is a modification of Rosenthal's (1983, p. 6) definition of family ritual which in turn is based upon the pioneering work of Bossard and Boll, who conducted extensive sociological research in the area of daily ritual (Bossard, 1948; Bossard and Boll, 1950). It is also consistent with concepts associated with ritual in anthropology (see the introduction to Chapter Six in this volume). Ritual is prescribed either by the participants themselves or by an authoritative person, institution, or tradition (e.g. a bishop, a church, a government, or the expectations of the culture). In the former case, a pattern of interaction develops which comes to be considered "the way a thing is to be done" (Bossard and Boll, 1950, p. 16). This is the way that many family rituals develop, such as those described in Elston-Hurdle and Poyzer (1989) and Spears (1990). In contrast, anthropologists often describe rituals which are prescribed by tradition, a prescription sometimes echoed by authoritative persons or institutions within the culture being studied (see Chapter Six in this volume).

By requiring human interaction before a repeated act can be considered to be a ritual, the definition which was used as a guide for this bibliography tends to exclude literature dealing with compulsive behaviors and other non-interactive behaviors of individuals (Rosenthal, 1983, p. 7). This focus on interaction is also consistent with the concept of ritual as communication discussed by Fischer (1973) and with the anthropological concept that rituals "dramatize a message" which is shared by the participants (Myerhoff, 1984, p. 306). Nevertheless, participants in a ritual may not be consciously aware of what its meaning is or what is being communicated. "Ritual is something to be done, not something to be thought out (Bossard and Boll, 1950, p. 9)

Although there is little in the nursing literature which deals directly with ritual behavior, many case presentations published for other reasons do include descriptions of rituals, especially those case presentations appearing in recent issues of *Nursing 89* and *Nursing 90*. Few of these deal with the elderly, however. This bibliography thus necessarily contains literature which covers a wide age range. Nevertheless, gerontological concerns are emphasized in the annotations. In addition, literature describing rituals involving young people often deals with concepts relevant to the elderly (e.g. grief, dying, loneliness, and hope).

In constructing this bibliography, a definition associated with family ritual was deliberately chosen in order to reflect the professional nurse's concern for family life and family process. Literature describing family rituals and issues thus constitutes an important group of entries in this bibliography (e.g. Francis, 1989; Furrh and Copley, 1989; Jack, 1988; Post, 1989; Prechtl, 1990; Shubin, 1990; Spears, 1990).

Some of the citations in this bibliography illustrate prescription of ritual by health care staff or by institutional policy. In a few of these cases the health care staff built upon a patient's past religious or family tradition in an attempt to individualize their approach to the care of the patient (e.g. Fish and Shelly,

1983; and Francis, 1989). More commonly however, the rituals were prescribed automatically for most patients in the setting. A number of articles illustrate that this last approach may have been helpful to some participants but inappropriate for others (e.g. Bayer, 1980; Mallison, 1985; Post, 1989). Although these rituals are quite different in origin and character than those which developed within the family, an occasional article in the bibliography deals with both kinds of ritual in a manner which highlights the contrast (e.g. Post, 1989).

In addition to the selections describing family interactions and those dealing with rituals emerging from institutional procedures, there are two other major categories of entries included in this bibliography: topical literature and transcultural literature. The topical entries deal with rituals related to reminiscing and reconciliation (e.g. Fournet, 1990; Kovach, 1990; Osborn, 1989), spiritual concerns and hope (e.g. Fish and Shelly, 1983; Miller, 1985; Weatherall and Creason, 1987), and loneliness and isolation (e.g. Kneisl, 1972; Rogers, 1989). Each of these topics have intrigued researchers from a wide variety of disciplines including gerontology, nursing, and social-psychology.

The transcultural category of entries includes two works by a nurse-anthropologist who has conducted ethnographic research and writes extensively about nursing issues from an anthropological perspective. (Leininger, 1970; Leininger, 1978). The descriptions of ritual found in both of these book chapters can be helpful in performing culturological assessments and in planning nursing interventions appropriate for transcultural situations.

References

Bossard, J.H.S. (1948). The sociology of child development. New York: Harper and Brothers.

Bossard, J.H.S., and Boll, E.S. (1950). Ritual in family living. Philadelphia: University of Pennsylvania Press.

Fischer, E. (1973). Ritual as communication. In J. Shaughnessy (Ed.), The roots of ritual. Grand Rapids, Michigan: William B. Eerdmans Publishing Company.

Myerhoff, B. (1984). Rites and signs of ripening: The intertwining of ritual, time, and growing older. In D.I. Kertzer and J. Keith (Eds.), Age and anthropological theory (pp. 305-330). Ithaca, N.Y.: Cornell University Press. (This work is annotated in Chapter Six of this volume).

Rosenthal, G. (1983). Family ritual and its relationship to family environment. Unpublished M.A. thesis, University of Connecticut.

ANNOTATED BIBLIOGRAPHY

5-1. Bayer, M. (1980). Saying goodbye through graffiti. <u>American Journal of Nursing</u>, <u>80</u>, 271.

This article describes the development of a ritual which took place upon the discharge of each client from a general hospital's short term (7-14 days) psychiatric unit in Augusta, Maine. As discharge approached, staff and patients cooperated in the construction of a "graffiti poster" by arranging pictures, titles, and cartoons clipped from periodicals in such a way as to convey affectionate and otherwise meaningful messages to the client being discharged. These posters were presented in a ceremony held just prior to discharge in which patients and staff gathered around the poster, read its messages together, and said their "good-byes".

This article could have been enhanced by the inclusion of relevant scholarly references and a discussion of possible meanings that such a ritual could have had for its participants. It could also have been enhanced by information and discussion regarding several questions which remain unanswered. Did the ritual continue or change after the author left her position as head nurse on the unit? Did the ritual function primarily as a rite of passage, a healing ritual, or both? If therapeutic, who were the primary beneficiaries, those who made the posters or those who were discharged? Nevertheless, the fact that questions such as these may be raised by reading the article makes it valuable for the planning of future research. In addition, it does function as a source of data concerning a rather interesting client-motivated ritual which was able to evolve in a health-care institution.

5-2. Carpenito, L.J. (1987). Spiritual distress. In L.J. Carpenito, <u>Nursing diagnosis: Application to clinical practice</u> (2nd ed.), (pp. 577-592). Philadelphia: J.B. Lippincott Company.

The intent of this chapter is to provide the nurse with some of the knowledge necessary to accurately diagnose and effectively treat patients experiencing spiritual distress. An introductory section contains a description of defining characteristics, risk factors, assessment criteria, and principles and rationale for nursing care associated with spiritual distress. A table providing an outline of major religious beliefs and practices associated with thirty-five Christian and non-Christian religious groups is also found in this section. This is followed by three sections providing assessment criteria, interventions, and outcome criteria specific to spiritual distress related to each of three etiologies-1) inability to practice spiritual rituals, 2) conflict between religious or spiritual beliefs and prescribed health regimen, and 3) crisis of illness, suffering, or death. This chapter provides valuable guidance to the practicing nurse who must deal with patients experiencing spiritual distress, although it is important for the practitioner to realize that the usefulness of the table of major religious beliefs and practices is limited because of its superficial nature and the diversity found within most of the listed religious groups. Since Carpenito is recognized within nursing as an expert on the topic of nursing diagnosis, this chapter should also be read by researchers interested in the current thinking within the nursing profession regarding appropriate ways of responding to a patient's religious rituals and spiritual concerns. Although the section most obviously relevant to researchers investigating ritual is "Spiritual Distress Related to Inability to Practice Spiritual Rituals," the other two sections are also of value since spiritual distress from these causes may influence a patient's ritual behavior.

5-3. Conrad, N.L. (1985). Spiritual support for the dying. Nursing Clinics of North America, 20, 415-426.

Based on nineteen nursing, pastoral, and psychological references as well as her own expertise as a consultant in Death Education and Nursing Education, the author focuses on nurses' recognition of spiritual needs and ways in which nurses may intervene in order to help patients meet some of those needs. The article begins with three short vignettes of terminally ill patients who participated in rituals and other activities consistent with their individual backgrounds (Jewish, Christian, and astrology). These are followed by a definition of spirituality and a discussion of spiritual needs and concepts such as the search for meaning, religious and secular conceptualizations of "god," the experience of hope, and the importance of spiritual care for professions subscribing to the idea of holistic client care. Specific approaches for assessing spiritual needs are also delineated as well as specific interventions for meeting these needs. The final major section of the article describes interdisciplinary collaboration in providing spiritual care.

Nurses and other care providers reading this article can benefit from its clear description of ways to help patients with their spiritual needs. Of particular interest for those investigating ritual behavior is the section on interventions which describes several secular and religious interpersonal rituals and other activities which clients may find helpful in meeting their spiritual needs.

5-4. Coolican, M., Vassar, E., and Grogan,J. (1989). Helping survivors survive. Nursing 89, 19, (8), 52-57.

The development and activities of the Trauma Support Team (T.S.T.) at Hartford Hospital are described in this article to provide insight into the emotional problems faced by the families of trauma victims and into some possible interventions through which their emotional needs can be met. Rituals of condolence and death anniversary contacts involving the family and representatives of the hospital are described as examples of such interventions. In gathering data needed to establish this multidisciplinary team, 150 families whose loved ones had died from trauma were asked to assess the care they received and how they might have been better supported. Among these data was the stated desire on the part of these families to see the victim as soon as possible and to spend time with him, practices now facilitated by the T.S.T., and practices which may permit parting rituals, rituals of affection, or other family rituals to be performed.

Although not enough information was presented to assess the generalizability of the survey data to other populations, this article provides useful information to program developers of other institutions. Researchers looking for examples of institutional ritual outreach to families and the facilitation of family ritual in health care institutions would also find this article to be of interest.

5-5. Elston-Hurdle, B.J. and Poyzer, D. (1989). Fighting over a critically ill patient. American Journal of Nursing, 89, 327-328.

This case presentation describes the impact of a family power struggle on the nursing care provided during the hospitalization of a 22 year old mother of two who was critically ill with a basilar artery thrombosis. Initially facing the conflicting demands of the patient's husband and mother, the nurses quickly took action aimed at helping to defuse the competition between these two strong-willed family members.

Although the major thrust of the article is to illustrate ways in which nurses may effectively deal with such situations, a few of the family behaviors illustrated are of interest to those investigating family ritual and its continuity, development, or re-emergence in times of stress. The article makes one wonder, for example, if behaviors such as the personal hygiene care which the mother insisted on providing with her special case of soaps and emollients was reflective of bathing rituals which had taken place 22 years earlier. If so, was such re-emergence a result of the stress itself; was it because of the dependant, infantile state of the patient; or was it because it was behavior rooted in an earlier time when the husband, the mother's present competition, was not around? This article could have been enhanced and made of greater value to the researcher with relevant references and a discussion of questions such as these.

5-6. Fish, S. and Shelly, J.A. (1983). The use of scripture. In S. Fish and J.A. Shelly (Eds.), Spiritual care: The nurse's role (2nd ed.), (pp. 117-134). Downers Grove, Ill.: InterVarsity Press.

As with the rest of this book, this chapter is intended to give guidance to nurses interested in enhancing their effectiveness in meeting their clients' spiritual needs. Utilizing six case examples mostly drawn from the experiences of nurses with medical-surgical patients in a large metropolitan hospital, the chapter provides suggestions concerning the appropriate timing, effective utilization, and cautions surrounding the use of scripture in providing meaningful nursing care to certain clients. Although written from the perspective of the Nurses Christian Fellowship and thus narrow in its specific focus, it would seem that some suggestions of this chapter can be generalized to meeting the needs of people of other faiths who make use of some form of written spiritual aids. The chapter is of value to those interested in interactive rituals related to serious illness because of the case examples illustrating the ritual use of scripture in ways that are seen by the authors as enhancing communication and the development of close interpersonal bonds between the nurse and hospitalized patient.

5-7. Fournet, K. (1990). Bonnie's love. Nursing 90, 20(9), 43.

This article presents a case study recounting the summer camp activities of a seven year old girl afflicted with pulmonary hypertension, a condition which predisposed her to infections, limited her activities, and led to her death four weeks after the end of camp. Interactions were described which involved acts of affection between this seriously ill child and her friends, and the intensive nature of her approach to the ritual of giving was highlighted.

While the author attributes these activities to the child's thoughtful and loving nature acquired under the influence of her parents, elements indicative of reconciliation can also be discerned in the description. Although reconciliation behaviors have been identified among the seriously and terminally ill in other studies, this article provides further indication of the breadth and variety of these behaviors.

5-8. Francis, B. (1989). What Jim found in his stocking. Nursing 89, 19(12), 112.

This short case presentation concerning a 48 year old rancher illustrates a situation in which nurses helped a patient overcome his feeling of hopelessness through an intervention which the patient found to be reminiscent of a meaningful childhood ritual. This patient had become a paraplegic as a result of a motor vehicle accident and was apparently discouraged over the impact of his condition on his ability to pursue his "lifelong dream" of ranching. Based upon the memories of his childhood which the patient had recounted to a nurse, a Christmas activity was planned to recreate events associated with his mother, a person whom he remembered as a major source of encouragement and strength.

The value of this article is lessened due to its lack of scholarly references. Nevertheless, it provides an interesting case example which can stimulate future research. The author attributes the efficacy of the activity to its ability to help the patient remember earlier significant events, yet such events had already been recounted to a nurse without obvious therapeutic effect. The researcher who reads this article may thus be led to raise questions regarding the psychological and other processes by which some rituals may have therapeutic effects which seem to exceed those of other behaviors related to reminiscence or remembering the past.

5-9. Francis, B. (1990). Walking the tightrope. Nursing 90, 20(2), 69.

This article describes the experience of an L.P.N. caring for a dying patient whose wife was vacillating in her decision concerning her husband's code status and whose doctor had recommended a "slow code" to "help his wife feel better." Although the thrust of this article was to note the emotional impact of this situation on the nurse involved, non-verbal family rituals taking place at the time of death were described. In addition, the reference to the proposed ritual of "slow code" was of interest for its potential to interfere with the capability of the family to be present at the time of death and thus carry out what they would consider to be appropriate parting rituals.

Although the use of limited anecdotal material to illustrate emotionally difficult nursing situations is appropriate, the article would be of greater interest if it contained additional material and further illustrations of family rituals which take place during such crises. Its value for ritual studies lies primarily in stimulating research questions related to two unstated issues raised by the presentation: 1) the potential interference of family ritual by the rituals of the health care staff, and 2) legal concerns surrounding staff rituals such as "slow codes".

5-10. Furrh, C.B. and Copley, R. (1989). One precious moment: What you can offer when a newborn infant dies. Nursing 89, 19(9), 52-54.

The purpose of this article is to recommend to maternity nurses specific ways in which they might more effectively meet the emotional needs of parents whose newborn infants have died. Most of the suggestions that are made involve nursing interventions specifically intended to allow parent/child rituals to develop or to encourage certain rituals which parents of living infants tend to perform. Several of these interventions involve facilitating interactions between the parents and the child's body, and making such interactions experiences which would likely lead to cherished memories. The ritual of sending home specific objects is also discussed.

Although the article lacks references which could provide an added degree of credibility to the suggestions, the professional credentials of at least one of the authors appears to be appropriate for the subject matter discussed. This article should not only be of interest to maternity nurses, but other nurses as well. Some of the suggestions made regarding the shaping of hospital activities in order to facilitate family ritual should be considered, in modified form, when caring for families of patients of any age who have died.

5-11. Jack, M. (1988). Something missing. Canadian Nurse, 84 (11), 21.

This article is a case description expressing the author's perception of events which took place during the last three hospitalizations of her terminally ill mother. As a nurse, the author was able to understand the physical changes which took place in her mother and the physical care which was given; as a family member she experienced distress due to the staff's ineffective communication with the family and behaviors which she attributed to a lack of compassion and sensitivity. Drawing upon her experiences as a professional and as a consumer, the author is able to offer the reader many suggestions for improved nursing care of the families of the terminally ill. For the scholar interested in family ritual, the article briefly describes some of the ritual behaviors which took place at the bedside and refers to the illness-caused disruptions to family mealtime and other "daily routines" which may have involved ritual.

Although the value of this article would be greater had the author included some scholarly references helpful in interpreting the events which took place, the article does lead the reader to reflect on the possibility that some of the upsetting staff behaviors described may in fact have had characteristics of ritual which performed some psychological or other function for the staff (e.g. the describing of the patient's markedly swollen head using the phrase "some swelling", the marching into the room in groups of two or three to ask the family to leave when they "repositioned mom"). This article thus alerts the researcher to the possibility of investigating health-care institutions as sub-cultures whose members act out rituals consistent with the sub-cultural norms of the institution and health-care professionals. If conflict were found to exist between the rituals or norms of the institutional sub-culture and the expectations or activities of patient families, such findings would help to explain the author's feeling that "Disapproval surrounded us; we were not behaving in the accepted manner."

5-12. Kneisl, C.R. (1972). Thoughtful care of the dying. In R.N. Browning and E.P. Lewis (Compilers), The dying patient: A nursing perspective (pp. 148-156). New York: The American Journal of Nursing Company.

"Cultural taboos, hospital rituals, and professional defense mechanisms all operate to make withdrawal from the dying patient a common behavior for personnel" (p. 148). Utilizing the findings of seventeen sociological studies, nursing studies, and other scholarly works, this chapter documents the existence of this behavior, discusses explanations for it, and suggests ways in which nursing care could be modified in order to lessen the sense of loneliness, isolation, and abandonment which the dying patient may be experiencing.

Although some of the examples of avoidance which are described by the author are now commonly recognized in nursing as practices to avoid, many of the examples may still be observed today. Researchers investigating hospital based rituals should thus read this chapter in order to glean ideas as to the kinds of behaviors which may be fruitful to investigate, the history of some present day hospital rituals, and, by comparison with more recent data, changes which may have taken place in nursing practice as rituals fall by the wayside or evolve into new forms. In addition, the cultural taboos mentioned in the chapter as explanations of staff avoidance rituals can provide insight into avoidance behaviors which may be observed among the friends and family of people who are dying or terminally ill.

5-13. Kovach, C.R. (1990). Promise and problems in reminiscence research. Journal of Gerontological Nursing, 16(4), 10-14.

Twenty nine studies are reviewed in this article in order to present what is currently known about reminiscence and the current state of reminiscence research. It is noted that although there is some evidence that reminiscence can have beneficial effects for some elderly, much of the research findings on reminiscence appear to be contradictory and inconsistent. Methodological limitations of the studies reviewed are discussed and some of the inconsistencies in research findings are attributed to these limitations, particularly to the lack of precision and agreement among scholars in defining and operationalizing what is meant by reminiscence.

The value of this article to those studying reminiscence as a ritual behavior in the elderly lies in the methodological issues it raises as well as in the directions for future research that it suggests. The call for studies linking reminiscence with other concepts such as "situationally derived needs" is of particular interest for those studying reminiscence and other rituals that may be related to situations such as illness, death, or institutionalization.

5-14. Lappe, J.M. (1987). Reminiscing: The life review therapy. Journal of Gerontological Nursing, 13(4), 12-16.

This article presents an experimental study which investigated the effect of participation in group reminiscing sessions on the self-esteem of elderly nursing home residents. Seventy-three female and ten male residents were recruited from four long-term care institutions in a mid-western city and randomly assigned to participate in either a reminiscence group or a current events discussion group within their facility. Half of each type of group met once a week for the ten week duration of the study and the other half of the groups met twice a week. All subjects were rated utilizing a previously validated self-esteem scale during the first session of their respective group and again within 24 hours of the final session. It was found that participants in the reminiscence groups had a significantly greater increase in self-esteem scores than those who were in the current events groups.

This study's findings make it of particular value in lending support to the concept of utilizing reminiscence therapy with groups of elderly. The author points out that "Although there is much written regarding reminiscing groups, a search of the literature revealed that no studies have compared the psychological benefits of a reminiscing group to another type of group to determine whether it is the group process alone or the reminiscing as an intervention that produces the effect." In addition, nurses and others interested in employing reminiscing as a therapeutic intervention should read this article for its review concerning the positive effects of reminiscing for the elderly and the practical guidance it gives in how to implement its use therapeutically. Ideas for future research concerning the effects of ritualized reminiscence may also be stimulated by reading this article. For example- are the benefits which have been attributed to group reminiscence in this and other studies primarily a result of each member having had a chance to tell his or her own story, or is there also a major effect related to the act of listening to other elderly tell their stories?

5-15. Leininger, M. (1970). The cultural context of behavior: Spanish-Americans and nursing care. In M. Leininger (Ed.), Nursing and anthropology: Two worlds to blend (pp. 111-127). New York: John Wiley and Sons.

By utilizing data specific to one particular sub-cultural group, this chapter provides an understanding of the cultural context of human behavior so that health personnel reading it may be encouraged to take an in-depth view of each of their patients and to "tailor-make" their plans of treatment in ways that would be appropriate for a patient's culturally based beliefs and practices. Ideas expressed in this selection by its nurse/anthropologist author were based upon nine anthropological, nursing, and other references as well as her own three years of anthropological research with Spanish-speaking families in semi-rural and urban areas of Colorado.

After a brief introduction to the concept of the cultural context of behavior and to some general aspects of Spanish-American culture, the author presents social, kinship, religious, political, and economic features of Spanish-American society. Much attention is paid to Spanish-American health/illness systems as well as to the nursing implications of the elements of Spanish-American culture presented. Of special interest to the scholar investigating ritual behaviors are the discussions of Spanish-American theories of illness causation and cure, discussions of specific folk beliefs such as mal ojo (evil eye) and maleficio (witchcraft), and some of the discussions related to suggested nursing interventions, such as the integration of ritualized health practices into the nursing care. In addition, the discussion of the Spanish-American cultural context can help the reader recognize meanings which may be associated with the rituals practiced by some Spanish-Americans. Lastly, this chapter is of value for any nurse who has certain sub-cultural groups of Spanish-Americans within his or her patient population and who wishes a better understanding of their cultural heritage.

5-16. Leininger, M. (1978). Culturological assessment domains for nursing practices. In M. Leininger (Ed.), Transcultural nursing: concepts, theories, and practices (pp. 85-106). New York: John Wiley and Sons.

The purpose of this chapter is to provide nurses with a rationale, some guiding principles, and some of the tools necessary to perform culturological assessments of their clients. Utilizing eleven anthropological, nursing, and other resources, and operating under the premise that "people have a right to have their cultural values, beliefs, and practices understood, respected, and considered" when receiving nursing care (p. 85), the author discusses nine culturological domains for assessment. Of particular interest for those involved in ritual studies are four of these domains: 1) Cultural Taboos and Myths, 2) Cultural Diversities, Similarities, and the Variations, 3) Life-Caring Rituals and Rites of Passages, and 4) Folk and Professional Health-Illness Cultural Systems. These sections point the reader toward assessing taboos and other aspects of a person's culture which may have ritualized components, such as eating behaviors and folk health care practices. In addition, they raise the consciousness of the nurse concerning highly ritualized aspects of modern nursing and health care which may be helpful to the client or act as a barrier to the practice or development of rituals meaningful to the client. This chapter is a valuable beginning resource for both the practitioner and researcher interested in ritual and/or cross cultural assessment.

5-17. Mallison, M.B. (1985). Urine testing: Ritual with no reason. American Journal of Nursing, 85, 13-14.

This brief article reports the findings of a retrospective chart audit conducted by J. Eisch and C. Driscoll in conjunction with the Robert Wood Johnson Foundation Teaching Nursing Home Program. They found considerable staff time devoted to glucose testing of the urine of 34 patients in an Health Related Facility and 24 patients in a Skilled Nursing Facility. They also found "no consistency in urine testing and no indication that the information was used." Although the article points out that it is customary to do procedures aimed at tight control of blood sugar levels in younger diabetic patients, physiologic evidence is noted which raises questions regarding the value of urine glucose testing for nursing home elderly. It is also noted that there is an absence in the literature of studies evaluating the efficacy of this and other procedures related to the management of diabetes in nursing home elderly.

Some of the questions raised by this article are left unanswered for the reader to ponder and perhaps attempt to answer with future research, e.g. "In monitoring, what are we trying to do and why?" Although one gets the impression that the author expects a physical care or physiologic answer to the question "why," the question and thus the article can stimulate many research questions in the mind of readers interested in ritual studies. Instead of asking the title question of the article, "Ritual with no reason?" one might ask, "What are the reasons (meanings) behind the ritual of such urine testing?" or, "What function does this ritual perform for the staff which has encouraged its continuation?" Possible answers to be explored in future research might include 1) it fosters a feeling of doing something worthwhile in the face of hopelessness, 2) it gives the staff a sense of connectedness with health-care providers and procedures of acute care settings which are seen as more normative, or 3) it provides a sense of connectedness with the past since such testing may have been a long term practice of the institution. Importantly, reading this article may stimulate researchers to ask if there are other nursing procedures being performed with minimal justification because of some value that the ritual has for the staff?

5-18. McCann, M.E. (1989). Sexual healing after heart attack. American Journal of Nursing, 89, 1132-1140.

Many people experience decreased sexual activity after a heart attack. Utilizing information from 17 references as well as her own professional experience, the author discusses a variety of psychological and sociological explanations for this phenomenon as well as the lack of physiologic justification for it in the majority of cases. Research findings presented can be of value to the nurse in counselling clients regarding specific techniques and other aspects of post infarction intercourse and alternative sexual activity.

The article can also provide research ideas to those investigating rituals related to serious illness. Some of the preparation and fore play activities discussed appear to be likely candidates for developing into ritual behaviors. Likewise, comparing these and other aspects of the mating ritual of post infarction patients with the behaviors of those who have not experienced myocardial infarctions is an area where only limited clinical research has already been done.

5-19. Miller, J.F. (1985). Inspiring hope. <u>American Journal of Nursing</u>, <u>85</u>, 22-25.

This review article utilizes 21 nursing, psychological, and other references in order to discuss the concept of hope, its importance for health, and ways of increasing it in patients who are seriously ill. The article begins by defining hope. The author next presents a section on "Diagnosing Hopelessness" in which various assessment strategies are suggested, including the modification of a quantitative instrument from the psychological literature. Most of the article is devoted to "Hope-Inspiring Strategies," such as promoting the patient's use of pre-existing support systems and the patient's development of goals and effective coping behaviors. Of interest is the emphasis on sustaining interpersonal relationships and the facilitation of conversation themes and ritual interactions meaningful to the patient. For patients whose hope has previously had its roots in "faith in God," the author discusses approaches and difficulties related to promoting religious ritual and other aspects of religion. Rituals which would have the effect of maximizing the aesthetic experience of the patient are also discussed.

Underlying the approaches recommended in this article is the concept that hope should not be understood as being restricted to "hope for a cure" but rather should include hope to reach one's full potential as a person. The author also believes "Hope doesn't necessarily spring eternal - sometimes it has to be carefully mined and channeled" (p. 23). This assumption, that hope can be increased by outside interventions, is obviously consistent with the general assumption of the healing professions that interventions can make a difference. What is less clear is whether imposed, suggested, or encouraged rituals would have the desired effect, even if freely developed rituals were elsewhere shown to be associated with increased hope. More research in ritual studies must be done in order to validate the effectiveness of some of the interventions suggested in this article.

5-20. Murphy, P. (1990). Helping Joanne die with dignity. Nursing 90, 20(9), 45-49.

This article presents a case study illustrating the nursing interventions which facilitated the death of a lady suffering from amyotrophic lateral sclerosis, a degenerative disease which can lead to total paralysis of a fully alert and mentally competent person. Soon to be "locked inside her body with no way to communicate with those she loved," the patient requested that she be disconnected from her life supports so that she would die. The major events recounted by this article illustrate family support for the decision, the resistance of the medical community, the legality of the procedure in the patient's home state (New Jersey), and the effectiveness of the described actions of nurses and organized nursing in overcoming the practical barriers to facilitating this death. The case study approach utilized in this article is appropriate for illustrating difficulties which may be faced by families in such situations and ways nurses may assist.

Although the emotional pro-nursing tone of the article tends to obscure the complexity of some of the moral issues involved, information is presented which raises such issues for the discerning reader. Of special interest is an accompanying insert describing federal and state court cases establishing the legal basis for these actions. In addition, the numerous parting rituals and rituals of affection described as having taken place among family and friends on the day the patient chose to die provides worthwhile reading for anyone interested in studying rituals related to death.

5-21. Osborn, C.L. (1989). Reminiscence: When the past eases the present. Journal of Gerontological Nursing, 15(10), 6-12.

The purpose of this article is to promote the therapeutic use of reminiscence groups in gerontological nursing. Thirty-nine scholarly references are utilized in discussing the value of reminiscence for the elderly, advantages of doing such reminiscence in group settings, and techniques which can be useful in establishing, maintaining, and leading such structured groups of elderly.

The value of this article for ritual studies is two fold: (1) it promotes an understanding of the phenomenon of gerontological reminiscence in general and thus may be helpful to scholars seeking to understand reminiscence as a ritual behavior of some elderly, and (2) it lists suggested topics for discussion in reminiscence groups, some of which, if pursued in such groups or in individual interviews, would clearly tend to involve descriptions of family ritual behaviors which may be of interest to the investigator (e.g. family traditions, proper manners, feeding the family). Researchers interested in these aspects of gerontological ritual would thus benefit from reading this well written and informative article.

5-22. Post, H. (1989). Letting the family in during a code. Nursing 89, 19(3), 43-46.

Allowing family members to be present during a code is not a common practice in American hospitals. The author describes this practice at a Michigan hospital and the events which led up to the adoption of the policy which now permits it. Other than a few references to parting rituals practiced by families at the time of their loved one's death, this article provides little insight into the family rituals which occur during serious illness or at the time of death.

Nevertheless, it should be read by those interested in investigating such rituals since it provides insight into the barriers to these rituals erected by most hospitals. Those investigating the rituals of health care providers would likewise find this article to be of interest since the reader gets the impression that the common practice of family exclusion is a ritual performed for the benefit of the staff. Lastly, those involved in policy decision making at hospitals should read this article since it discusses the benefits the family may derive from being present, the increased stress experienced by the staff when the family is allowed to be present, and, in an accompanying legal opinion, legal benefits from instituting such a policy.

5-23. Prechtl, A. (1990). The strength of Hank's love. Nursing 90, 20(5), 192.

This is a short anecdote of a nurse's emotional response to the death of a patient with Alzheimer's Disease. Its intent is to illustrate what the author sees as the positive effects that the husband's love for his wife had upon his wife's condition and upon the nurse's ability to respond with feeling.

Although this causal relationship remains unproven, the article is of interest for its description of several rituals which took place between this patient and her husband after her admission to a nursing home. Particularly noteworthy is her participation in displays of affection involving touch in ways similar to those reported elsewhere for patients who are not mentally debilitated. By reading this article, scholars may be stimulated to develop research questions related to comparing the ritual behaviors of families who have a mentally debilitated member with those of families who do not.

5-24.   Rogers, B.L. (1989). Loneliness: Easing the pain of the hospitalized elderly. Journal of Gerontological Nursing, 15(8), 16-21.

The purpose of this study was to explore the incidence of loneliness and factors related to it in patients on a medical/family practice unit in a large, urban, mid-western, acute care hospital. A convenience sample consisted of 31 medically competent, English speaking patients who were 55 years old or older and hospitalized for two days or more. They were interviewed using an instrument designed to identify some of the types of objects and persons to which they felt emotionally attached and to assess the degree of this attachment. It also assessed the degree of their separation from significant objects and persons as well as the extent of the loneliness that the respondents were experiencing. The reliability and validity of this instrument were reported to have been established in several previous studies.

Likert scale and short answer items revealed that the patients sampled tended to have a moderately high degree of emotional investment in a variety of persons and objects and had loneliness scores averaging in the moderate range. Content analysis of responses to open ended questions revealed considerable distress due to separation from certain persons, things, or activities.

Although characteristics of the sample and sample selection process limit the generalizability of the findings, this article contributes to the knowledge base concerning loneliness in hospitalized adults, a topic that the author indicates has been minimally researched. It is also of interest to researchers in ritual studies because of the ideas that it may stimulate. The author acknowledged that a patient's loneliness may be exacerbated by his experiencing "disruptions in familiar patterns of activity and interaction" (p. 16). Nevertheless, other than mentioning general categories such as "recreation" and "entertainment," she identified objects and people missed without describing rituals and other patterns of interaction which were associated with them. It would seem that the patient may have attached special meaning or significance to the interactions in addition to the non-interacting object or person. This study can thus be expanded by a researcher in ritual studies in order to explore more thoroughly the experience of the hospitalized elderly.

5-25. Ross, H.K. (1990). Lessons of life. Geriatric Nursing, 11, 274-275.

This article presents an unusual twist to the investigation of the phenomenon of life review. In contrast to the frequently discussed topics of the usual beneficial effects of life review upon the elderly who do it, Ross has investigated effects upon the listeners. Twenty-five nurses, social workers, and mental health aides enrolled in a geriatric training program conducted a series of interviews with elderly persons during which a structured outline was utilized to stimulate the elderly person to recount events experienced throughout the lifespan. Students also kept a record of their own reactions, feelings, and outlook toward the persons interviewed and these were shared during in-class discussions. As the interviews progressed, these records included less negative descriptors and indicated increased understanding of the elders' experiences and strengths. In addition, the students' attitudes toward the elderly and aging seemed to develop through a series of seven steps culminating in "a hope to transfer their new-found outlook into improved care of elderly patient."

Nurses and nurse educators concerned with professional attitudes toward and perceptions of the elderly would benefit from reading this article in order to gather ideas concerning the possible benefits of incorporating a similar activity into their own practice or educational program. In addition, this article can stimulate a variety of research ideas for those interested in reminiscing as a social ritual involving interaction and response. For example- what is the effect on family members who may listen to their older members ritually tell their story over and over again as a part of the life review process? Do they experience a series of changes as did Ross's students?

5-26. Shubin, S. (1990). Offer families hope. . . or help them let go. Nursing 90, 20(3), 44-49.

This article uses a case presentation format to illustrate and discuss a variety of issues related to the nursing care of the families of traumatic brain injury patients. After a brief description of the clinical situation, the article presents two contrasting descriptions of events which had taken place during the institutionalization of a 22 year old female who had entered a persistent vegetative state following an automobile accident three weeks prior to her scheduled wedding day. Although the major emphasis of the article is on the contrasting perceptions of the family and hospital staff regarding the etiology of the many reported instances of miscommunication between these two groups of people, several instances of family ritual and routinized care are mentioned. The contrasts in meaning attributed to these behaviors by the two groups illustrate the need for further knowledge on the part of health care professionals so that they might better interpret the behaviors of their patients' families. One also wonders if some of the instances of miscommunication which are reported may have been the result of ritualized behaviors on the part of health care personnel. Consequently, this article should be read by those interested in identifying hospital based rituals, the meaning of rituals, or ideas for research into the impact of nursing ritual behavior on the quality of care.

5-27. Sodestrom, K.E. and Martinson, I.M. (1987). Patients' spiritual coping strategies: A study of nurse and patient perspectives. Oncology Nursing Forum, 14, 41-46.

The purposes of this exploratory study were to describe the spiritual coping strategies of patients hospitalized with cancer, to assess their nurses' awareness of these strategies, and to determine the level of agreement between patients and nurses in identifying the coping strategies utilized. Interviews were conducted separately with a convenience sample of twenty-five nurses from an oncology unit of a major medical center and with one randomly selected patient of each nurse. These interviews utilized a survey questionnaire adapted from a spiritual coping instrument described in a 1981 unpublished manual of data collection instruments from the University of Washington. Data indicated that families, friends, clergy, nurses, and physicians were all utilized at various frequencies by the patients for spiritual coping. Nurses correctly identified the patients' reliance upon these resource persons less than 60% of the time. Of interest for those investigating interpersonal ritual is that 64% of the patients reported asking others to pray with them and 56% read the Bible, some of whom, the authors noted, may have required the help of others due to failing vision. Few spiritual activities had been noted by nurses, however.

Although the authors are correct in pointing out that the descriptive nature of this study and its small sample size limit its generalizability, this article remains of value to researchers in ritual studies for the coping rituals that it identifies. Nurses may also benefit from reading it because of the suggestions for improved nursing care that it contains.

5-28. Spears, J.B. (1990). Until death do us part. Nursing 90, 20(5), 45.

This vignette shows the difficulties experienced by a nurse in caring for her husband while he was terminally ill with late-stage Hodgkin's disease. Although few rituals are mentioned in the account, there are some illustrations of routinized communications over a distance during the periods of time that the patient required protective isolation.

This is one of the few nursing articles describing such home based family rituals of children in the face of terminal illness. It is of further interest because the reported impact of the illness on the sleeping routine of the children calls attention to the shortage elsewhere in the nursing literature of descriptions of bedtime rituals of families facing terminal illness.

5-29. Weatherall, J., and Creason, N.S. (1987). Validation of the nursing diagnosis, spiritual distress. In A.M. McLane (ed.), Classification of nursing diagnoses: Proceedings of the seventh conference North American Nursing Diagnosis Association (pp. 182-185). St. Louis: The C.V. Mosby Company.

This study was intended to validate the defining characteristics of the nursing diagnosis of spiritual distress which have been accepted by the North American Nursing Diagnosis Association (NANDA). Utilizing a content analysis of 34 relevant nursing articles printed between 1959 and 1984 as well as data from the nursing records of 13 patients (seven females and six males) ranging in age from 22-92 years old, 464 cues were identified as indicating that a patient had spiritual needs or required spiritual care. More than 60% of these cues were seen as supporting the 24 NANDA defining characteristics of spiritual distress.

Of particular interest for ritual studies is that the characteristic "unable to choose or chooses not to participate in usual religious practices" was supported as a valid indicator of spiritual distress by the patient data and to a lesser extent by the nursing literature. From a gerontological perspective it is interesting to note that all the patients displaying this characteristic were over 55 years old.

The authors indicate that applications of this study are limited by the small size of the patient sample and by the reliability of the content analysis procedures utilized. Unfortunately, the article gives no indication of what these procedures were. Nevertheless, it remains of peripheral interest to those interested in ritual studies because one commonly accepted etiology of spiritual distress, the separation from religious/cultural ties, can include ties involving ritual. Similarly, "cues having to do with relationships with others" was identified as one of the five most "clinically useful" categories of defining characteristics, a category which would seem to encompass interpersonal ritual cues. By reading this article, a nurse researcher interested in interpersonal rituals may thus be encouraged to investigate further the relationship between such ritual cues and the experience of spiritual distress.

5-30. Wilson, V.C. and Jacobson E. (1990). How can we dignify death in the I.C.U. American Journal of Nursing, 90(5), 38-42.

The purpose of this article is to describe ways in which I.C.U. nursing care can be modified in order to increase the dying patient's control over his care and care decisions. This article begins with a description of three deaths which occurred in an I.C.U. and which illustrate the importance of clear communication between the recipients and providers of health care services. Physician reluctance to discontinue treatment when requested to do so and the de-emphasis on pain control and interpersonal communication in favor of "medical management" were also noted. The discussion which follows provides the reader with specific suggestions as to ways in which nurses could fulfil their role as patient advocates by facilitating communication between family and physicians, by encouraging the physicians to assess the ability to achieve their goals, and by suggesting alternatives to the medical care which is being provided.

This article is of value to nurses needing guidance in how to approach similar situations whether in the I.C.U. or in other areas of an acute care facility. Other readers can gain insight into some of the rituals of the health care system as well as some of the barriers it erects to family ritual when death is near.

6

RITUALS RELATED TO DEATH, DYING AND SERIOUS INFIRMITY: AN ANTHROPOLOGICAL BIBLIOGRAPHY

Robert D. Woodcock

INTRODUCTION

This bibliography describes a selection of anthropological studies and theoretical papers which will be helpful to researchers from many disciplines who are interested in investigating rituals related to serious illness and death. Anthropologists tend to study the structure and characteristics of communities of people, including their customs, languages, literature, myths, and beliefs. From an anthropological perspective, a ritual must thus be understood as taking place within the context of a particular community of people.

Rituals are not just repetitive acts, but prescribed sequences of events which have meaning and purpose for the community in which they are performed. These concepts are consistent with those which were utilized to guide the formation of the nursing bibliography in the previous chapter (see introduction to Chapter Six). Anthropological studies often describe rituals which have developed over many generations and have become prescribed by tradition, a prescription sometimes echoed by authoritative persons or institutions within the culture being studied. Studies of modern communities have identified rituals with a shorter developmental history (e.g. Gubrium, 1975; Ross, 1977). Some of these rituals may have been developed by the very people observed by the researcher in a way similar to some of the family and institutional rituals examined in annotations found in the preceding chapter.

There is an expectation in anthropology that rituals carry some meaning for the participant. "Ritual refers to the sequence of events that are performed; their context and connotation gives them meaning and purpose" (du Toit, 1980, p. 28). Nevertheless, some participants might not be conscious of these meanings nor be able to verbalize them to the anthropologist.

Myerhoff (1984) provides a description of some of the important functions of ritual for the members of a community.

"Because rituals dramatize a message about continuity, predictability, and tradition, they are inherently connective, providing integration of several kinds: of the self with itself as it contemplates its movement through biological and historical change; of the self with the culture, by the use of familiar, often axiomatic common symbols; of the self with others, joining celebrants into an often profound community where all manner of distinctions may be transcended in an all-embracing, sacred unity." (Myerhoff, 1984, p. 306)

It is worthwhile to point out that the "sacred unity" which rituals may promote is sometimes viewed not only as a unity which is sacred but as a unity with the sacred, with the divine. In addition, the connective and integrative power of ritual can transcend time, changing the participants perception of time and promoting a communion with those who have gone before and those yet to come. Rites of passage may especially promote a change in a person's relationship to others in time, space, and the social order. The relationship of ritual and time is explored at some length in two of the theoretical papers included in this bibliography (Myerhoff, 1984; Humphreys, 1981).

In many societies, old people have special roles in rituals. Not the least of these is the role of expert in ritual performance and interpretation. In addition, the elderly may find ritual to be especially significant because of the discontinuities in life they are likely to have experienced (Keith, 1990, p. 99)

"Ritual is a form by means of which culture presents itself to itself... It allows old people in particular to present claims regarding their vanished past and proof of their continuing existence and honor." (Myerhoff, 1984, p. 320).

Ritual is thus a particularly appropriate topic for inclusion in a gerontology publication.

Anthropologists engage in a variety of research activities which collectively can be described as doing ethnography or utilizing the ethnographic approach. Often, these activities have included participating in ancient ceremonies, observing day to day behavioral patterns, analyzing written or oral texts, and conducting informal interviews. Whatever specific research activities are employed in a given situation, the major aspect of the research which makes it ethnographic is that the researcher approaches these tasks in a way which seeks to reveal the culture being studied from the perspective of those who are members of that community. Although others would use the phrase "the ethnographic approach" somewhat more broadly than does Ragucci (1990), it is reasonable that she uses the term "participant-observation" as being synonymous with "the ethnographic approach" (p. 167). When doing ethnography, the observer or researcher is in some sense participating in the culture, and, to an extent, acquiring an insider's understanding of the world and the various meanings that the experiences of life have for the members of the community being studied.

The selections incorporated into this bibliography can be categorized into three major groups: literature describing death ritual, literature related to healing and health care, and theoretical literature. Rituals related to death and dying have figured very prominently in anthropological literature. By studying them, one might begin to understand the religion of a culture. Mandelbaum (1965) suggests that death rituals fit into, reflect, and reinforce cultural themes and so provide a useful way to begin to understand a culture and the people who make up a cultural group. Five of the studies included in this bibliography describe some of these important rituals (Badone, 1989; Glaser and Strauss, 1965; Gubrium, 1975; Humphreys, 1981; Mandelbaum, 1965).

The bibliography includes three studies which describe healing rituals conducted by members of specific cultural groups: Black South Africans (du Toit, 1980), Navaho (Kluckhohn and Leighton, 1962), and certain sub-cultural groups in Peru (Joralemon, 1986). Articles which discuss rituals involving residential and health care institutions and their personnel have also been included because of their particular interest to the nurse researcher investigating ritual (Glaser and Strauss, 1965; Gubrium, 1975; Leininger, 1978; Ross, 1977).

Other selections in the bibliography describe characteristics of ritual from a theoretical perspective, addressing issues such as the relationship between aging and ritual, the connective and integrative functions of ritual, and the relationship between ritual, death, and time (e.g. Humphreys, 1981; Keith, 1990; Myerhoff, 1984). Two theoretical papers from nursing publications are included which discuss the ethnographic approach and its usefulness in both nursing and anthropological research (Cameron, 1990; Ragucci, 1990). These entries, along with Dougherty and Tripp-Reimer (1985), provide a theoretical link between the disciplines of anthropology and nursing which are represented in this bibliography and the one in Chapter 5 of this volume.

ANNOTATED BIBLIOGRAPHY

6-1. Badone, E. (1989). Religion and death I: Orthodox models and local interpretations. In E. Badone, The Appointed Hour (pp.158-188). Berkeley: University of California Press.

The book The Appointed Hour is a report of a study based on 15 months of anthropological field work during 1983-1984 in two Breton communities, Plouguerneau and La Feuille. Chapter Six, "Religion and Death I: Orthodox Models and Local Interpretations," builds upon the work of many other scholars as well as discussing the author's own findings concerning Breton beliefs, festivals, and folk rituals related to death and dying. The last section of this chapter puts these findings in the historical perspective of pre-Christian influences and the influences of the seventeenth century and twentieth century Catholic missions, influences which the author sees as having helped elevate death to a dominant motif in Breton society. Little is mentioned regarding the specific research methods utilized in this study but appropriate participant observer and interviewing techniques are implied.

Some of the death beliefs identified by Badone have roots in pre-Christian Celtic folk tradition. Likewise, the merging of Catholic and non-Christian folk elements in Breton religion can be seen in the rituals related to death and the dead that the author describes as taking place on three festival days, the most important of which is Toussaint (All Saints' Day). This festival apparently surpasses Christmas, Easter, and New Year's Day in the level of participation and excitement generated.

From the standpoint of those investigating family ritual rather than public ritual, the section on "Folk Rituals for the Dying" is particularly interesting. Several rituals reported in this section are performed in order to aid the dying, not in the Catholic sense of spiritual preparation for the afterlife, but with the intent of helping the person escape suffering by speeding up the dying process. Health professionals may also benefit from reading this section, not so much for the specific information it provides regarding a particular culture in northwestern France, but for its value as a concrete reminder that prolonging the life of the dying may not be a value which is held by the recipient of care and his or her family.

6-2. Cameron, C. (1990) The ethnographic approach: Characteristics and uses in gerontological nursing. Journal of Gerontological Nursing, 16(9), 5-7.

As the title indicates, this article discusses the characteristics of ethnographic research techniques and their usefulness in gerontological nursing. The author begins by citing several other scholars in order to present a brief introduction to the anthropological roots of ethnography, to what ethnographic research entails, and to possible applications in research concerning elderly health care needs. An hypothesis generating study which had been conducted by the author is then described in order to provide an example of ethnographic nursing research techniques in action.

Nursing scholars intent on describing rituals or other regularities and variations in human behavior can benefit greatly from reading this article as it clearly explains a methodology that is appropriate for such endeavors. In addition, the study presented in the article can serve as a model for future ethnographic nursing research.

6-3. Dougherty, M.C. and Tripp-Reimer, T. (1985). The interface of nursing and anthropology. Annual Review of Anthropology, 14, 219-41.

Utilizing 194 references, this chapter documents the contributions of the fields of nursing and anthropology to each other and discusses the differences between the nursing/anthropological interface and the medical/anthropological interface. Arguing for the existence of a "natural alliance," the authors point out similarities of the two fields in research topics, research methodologies, conceptual approaches, and the rooting of research problems in the "client perspective." Methodological differences which the authors see as resulting from nursing's "early" reliance on quantitative sociological models are also discussed. Although the chapter does not specifically address the topic of ritual behavior, other than a brief reference to "ritual and magic in practice" as a fruitful topic for academic inquiry, it is a thought provoking resource for researchers in either field who are preparing to investigate an aspect of human behavior that is within the domain of the other. Those investigating rituals or ritual changes which may be responses to actual or potential health problems would particularly benefit from reading this enlightening and well documented chapter.

6-4. du Toit, B.M. (1980). Religion, ritual, and healing among urban Black South Africans. Urban Anthropology, 9(1), 21-49.

This article describes a 1973 study which examined religious and healing beliefs and practices among Black residents of Durban, South Africa. Data indicate that neither active membership in a Christian church nor living in an urban area with access to modern medical facilities precludes traditional belief in the supernatural or the practice of traditional religious and other ritual. Ninety percent of the 432 persons interviewed were members of Christian churches, almost half of whom had attended church during the two weeks prior to the interview, and most visit a modern medical clinic and are served by medical doctors. Nevertheless, almost half reported receiving messages from an ancestral spirit, almost half performed traditional rituals for health and success, and many consulted with diviners when experiencing an illness or other crisis, especially when the illness or crisis was severe.

Interview data are supplemented with information gleaned from the 40 references cited as well as from the author's own anthropological expertise. The article begins with an introduction to concepts relevant to religion, ritual, and healing, including a discussion of assumptions which anthropologists sometimes hold regarding those topics. This is followed by a brief description of traditional religious beliefs and practices of Bantu-speaking peoples, an history of Christianization in the Durban area, and a rather extensive account of the meaning, utilization, and underlying belief systems of life cycle, protective, and healing rituals. Uses of herbalists, western medical specialists, and faith healers are also discussed. A table illustrates the utilization of a variety of health resources as a function of health status.

Little information is presented in the article concerning sample selection and interviewing technique. Interpretation of the data would have been enhanced had the author analyzed the data statistically to see if there were significant differences between groups with different religious affiliation or church attendance patterns in their maintenance of traditional practices. Nevertheless, this article is a valuable resource to researchers and clinicians alike. It provides much information concerning traditional rituals of a particular group of people as well as the impetus for researchers to examine various ethnic groups in other modern urban settings in order to identify possible continuations of traditional beliefs and behaviors. Reading this article can also serve as a reinforcement to clinicians' awareness that clients may pursue traditional remedies along with those of modern medicine.

6-5.   Glaser, B.G. and Strauss, A.L. (1965). The ritual drama of mutual pretense. In B.G. Glaser and A.L. Strauss, <u>Awareness of dying</u> (pp. 64-78). Chicago: Aldine Publishing Company.

In this chapter, the authors describe ritual interactions in U.S. hospital settings in which the dying person and his professional caregivers are aware of his impending death yet all act as if he were going to live. The data were collected through on-sight observation and interviewing, methodologies appropriate for identifying and describing ritual behavior in this and other cultures. Analogies with other pretending behaviors are drawn, the consequences and fragility of such arrangements are noted, and the rules of behavior which are followed during such ritual interactions are discussed.

Although the authors elsewhere in the book address issues surrounding the awareness of dying from a sociological perspective, this chapter raises anthropological issues by attributing the tendency of staff to participate in such behaviors to their status as "typical Americans." This chapter is thus not only valuable as a source of insight into a specific ritual related to dying which may take place between American patients and staff and, by extension, the patients' friends and family, it is also of value because of some interesting questions it raises for anthropological research. What other cultures, if any, practice rituals of mutual pretense and how are these rituals carried out? How has the American ritual changed since the authors did their research? Who is most likely to participate in such rituals- family, friends, health care staff, or other acquaintances of the patient?

6-6. Gubrium, J.F. (1975). Living and dying at Murray Manor. New York: St. Martin's Press.

Several chapters in this book deal with clientele and staff attitudes regarding death and dying, their characteristic modes of witnessing these events, and associated ritual behaviors observed by the author during a several month period as a participant observer at a residential facility for the aged referred to as Murray Manor. Similarities and differences were noted in the three separate "death worlds" of clientele, floor staff, and "top staff" and problems resulting from their interaction were discussed. These included differences in mode and ability to witness death and dying as well as modes of acquisition and attitudes toward "death news." Of particular interest is the discrepancy between the self reported research based beliefs of the "top staff" and their behaviors as observed by the author and perceived by the floor staff and clientele. This discrepancy is seen by the author as one example of the influence of "place" on death related behaviors. When in a location inhabited exclusively by "top staff," the "world at hand" influences them to assume clientele may appreciate death, an attitude consistent with the behaviors of clientele observed by the author. When in a location of mixed population, "top staff" exhibited behaviors strikingly discordant with these attitudes.

Few of the rituals performed by clientele were non-verbal behaviors, and only a few examples were given which indicated variations possibly resulting from differences in interpersonal bonds. Still, this can provide gerontologists with insights into the attitudes and verbal rituals which may typically occur between elderly acquaintances experiencing death or dying. It should also be read by facility administrators, nurses, and anyone concerned with staff behaviors in the face of death and dying. In addition, the discrepancies the author noted as apparently resulting from the influence of "place" should be of interest to all researchers in ritual studies as they point out the danger of relying solely upon reported behaviors and the value of utilizing the technique of participant observation.

6-7. Humphreys, S.C. (1981). Death and time. In S.C. Humphreys and H. King (Eds.), Mortality and immortality: The anthropology and archaeology of death (pp. 261-283). New York: Academic Press.

In this chapter, the author summarizes three aspects of the relationship between death and time in various cultures- 1) the culturally accepted "right time" to die, 2) death as a rite of passage requiring time for the transition, and 3) the nature of time in the world of the dead. The discussion surrounding death as a rite of passage makes this chapter of particular interest for ritual studies. In this most lengthy aspect of the chapter, the author describes social processes and rituals involved in "becoming dead," including the farewell greetings involving the dying, the ritual redistribution of roles and properties, the ritual of the disposal of the corpse, its replacement with a stable material representing the deceased (e.g. mummy, tombstone, ashes), and, ever so briefly, the behaviors of health care personnel when caring for the dying. By also illustrating that the English concept of the "moment of death" as a sharp demarcation separating a period of dying from being dead does not necessarily exist in all cultures, the author further emphasizes the social nature of this gradual transformation.

Unfortunately, the brevity of the text (18 pages) and the author's heavy reliance on illustrations from ancient Greece precludes a comprehensive presentation of all three of the selected aspects of the interrelationship of death and time which were discussed. Nevertheless, this chapter is of value for its extensive bibliography (57 references), for the overview that it provides of rituals and social processes related to dying, and for the encouragement it may provide to other researchers to study these phenomena which, according to the author, are under-researched and often too narrowly conceived.

6-8. Joralemon, D. (1986). The performing patient in ritual healing. Social Science Medicine, 23, 841-845.

This ethnographic study is based upon the author's observations of healing rituals performed by a curandero practicing in two distinct Peruvian coastal communities- one village six miles from an urban center which was the recipient of a large migration after the 1970 earthquake, and one agricultural community located further from the quake area. While the practitioner produced essentially the same ritual procedure in the two locations, the nature of the patient's involvement varied greatly. The villagers displayed more passive participation, while the members of the agrarian community were more actively engaged and willing to improvise at various points. Although the curandero attributes these differences to the relative inexperience of the villagers with the ritual, these differences were still evident during the third performance with the villagers.

The author attributes the differences to the differing social contexts from which the patients are drawn in the two locations and to an hypothesized reduced sense of self efficacy in the village population because of its experiences related to the earthquake and migration. Regardless of the cause of the population differences, the data from this study suggest that patients as well as the folk practitioners contribute to the ritual process, and that this patient contribution is as evident in the choice to remain passive in the therapeutic process as it is when active partnership with the practitioner is sought.

In spite of the uncertainty raised by the small sample (one practitioner) of the study, this article is of value because of the questions it stimulates for future research. Can the suggested influence of patients on the ritual process be validated by observations of other folk practitioners in other settings? Are similar processes taking place in the interaction of patients with modern medical healers and the treatments that occur? More specifically, is patient passivity with modern medical healers a result of practitioner style only, or is it in part, as the author suggests, an adaptation stimulated by the patient?

6-9. Keith, J. (1990). Age in social and cultural context: Anthropological perspectives. In R.H. Binstock and L.K. George (Eds.), Handbook of aging and the social sciences (3rd ed.), (pp. 91-111). San Diego: Academic Press, Inc.

Employing 169 references, this chapter reviews the research which has investigated social and cultural influences upon aging. Characteristics of social, cultural, and subjective contexts that influence the way persons experience old age and maintain well-being were identified and discussed along with proposed mechanisms by which some of these characteristics may have their effect upon the elderly. Great diversity in the significance and even the definition of age was also noted. As is common in anthropological literature, examples from a variety of cultures are offered throughout the chapter in order to illustrate the concepts being discussed.

The chapter is divided into three major parts. "Old People in Society" reviews the status, treatment, and experiences of elderly from a cross-cultural perspective, highlights gender differences, and discusses the relationship of the elderly to social change. The second major section discusses the interrelationship of "Aging and Culture," including the significant influence the aging have had in the evolution and the transmission of cultures as well as the influence which distinctive characteristics of a culture can have on the well-being and status of the elderly. The third major section, "Age in Society," traces aspects of three popular foci of ethnographic research- formal age systems, the creation of informal support networks and age-homogeneous communities, and the relationship of age to kinship and other principles of social organization.

Of particular interest to scholars in ritual studies is the discussion in the "Age and Culture" section regarding rituals and their significance for the elderly. The author briefly discusses a variety of topics such as sex differences regarding rites of passage into an older status, the relationship between ritual timing and the potential for conflict in society, ritual routes to social participation of the elderly, and the role of ritual in providing a sense of continuity during experiences of discontinuity. Although rituals related to illness or death were not specifically discussed, scholars interested in these topics would still benefit from reading this chapter because of the general concepts related to ritual that it discusses. The chapter is also of exceptional value to researchers interested in many other topics in anthropology and gerontology because of the extensive number of references it contains. Some researchers may also benefit from consulting Keith's earlier edition of this chapter which contains some additional detail concerning ritual and provides interesting insights into the developing relationship between the disciplines of anthropology and gerontology. (Keith, J. (1985). Age in Anthropological Research. In R.H. Binstock and E. Shanas (eds.), Handbook of Aging and the Social Sciences (2nd ed.), (pp. 231-263). New York: Van Nostrand Reinhold Co.)

6-10.   Kluckhohn, C. and Leighton, D. (1962). The supernatural: Things to do and not to do. In C. Kluckhohn and D. Leighton, The Navaho (rev. ed.), (pp. 200-223). Garden City, N.Y.: Doubleday and Company.

In this chapter, an anthropologist (Kluckhohn) and a physician (Leighton) describe some of the daily and special ceremonial rituals that Navahos practice with the intent of warding off dangers and establishing harmony between themselves and supernatural beings and powers. Along with the rest of the book, these descriptions are based upon previously published literature as well as the authors' own field work with the Navaho in conjunction with the Indian Education Research Project of the University of Chicago and the United States Office of Indian Affairs. After briefly illustrating taboos and avoidance behaviors, the authors present details of rituals consisting of positive actions and discuss the world view and beliefs which seem to underlie these practices. Separate sections on ceremonial music, sand painting, and divination are of interest in their own right as well as providing background for understanding the healing rituals and beliefs described toward the end of the chapter.

This chapter is of value for researchers seeking to identify rituals of the Navaho which may be practiced when they are faced with serious or terminal illness. Other researchers may find its bibliography of 30 references on the supernatural to be particularly useful. It should also be read by nurses and other practitioners who may be caring for Navaho patients so that traditional practices can be understood and institutional routines can be adjusted to permit desired rituals to be performed.

6-11.   Leininger, M. (1978). Two strange health tribes: the Gnisrun and Enicidem in the United States. In M. Leininger, Transcultural nursing:

Concepts, theories, and practices (pp. 267-281). New York: John Wiley and Sons.

Utilizing a style of presentation that is reminiscent of some anthropological descriptions of remote cultures, the author draws on the work of five other scholars as well as her own experience as a nurse and as an anthropologist in order to describe the professions of nursing and medicine as sub-cultures of American society. Since she recognizes that many readers may be members of these professions, their "tribal names" and other referent terms were changed (spelled backwards) to provide the reader with a further sense of remoteness and thus, hopefully, increased receptivity to the insights regarding the professions which are presented. Looking at each profession separately as well as from an interactional perspective, the author describes behaviors and ritual practices, beliefs, and changes over time which she feels would enhance the reader's understanding of the "dominant cultural features of the two tribes." (p. 268)

Since many of the rituals described are those involving professionals only (e.g. rites of passage, historic rituals of interaction between the professions), the direct usefulness of this chapter for those interested in identifying patient ritual is minimal. Nevertheless, the researcher may find this article helpful in providing an understanding of the cultural milieux which may surround patients and families attempting to practice their rituals in times of illness.

6-12. Mandelbaum, D.G. (1965). Social uses of funeral rites. In H. Feifel (ed.), The meaning of death (pp. 189-217). New York: McGraw-Hill.

In this chapter, an anthropologist describes the funerary rites of six cultures in order to illustrate what he sees as the social functions of these rituals and the psychological ambivalence of the participants which they reflect. Details concerning an interesting selection of the ritual behaviors of friends and family of the dying or deceased are interspersed among the descriptions of organized community ceremonies. Although many of the behaviors discussed are quite dissimilar in specific details, intercultural similarities are also noted. It is suggested that death rituals fit into, reflect, and reinforce cultural themes and that their study may therefore serve as a useful way to begin anthropological analysis of cultures and to understand the people who make up a cultural group. Reading this chapter may also stimulate scholars in sociology, psychology, and other fields to consider ways in which the study of rituals might enhance their understanding of some of the human phenomena which they are investigating. This chapter is of particular value to people already interested in identifying rituals related to death and dying because of the many ceremonial and interpersonal rituals described.

6-13. Myerhoff, B. (1984). Rites and signs of ripening: The intertwining of ritual, time, and growing older. In D.I. Kertzer and J. Keith (Eds.), Age and anthropological theory (pp. 305-330). Ithaca, N.Y.: Cornell University Press.

Like most of the chapters in this book, this chapter is based upon a presentation made at a 1981 workshop organized by the Behavioral Sciences Research Program of the National Institute on Aging. Utilizing 29 references as well as her own experience as an anthropologist, the author presents her theoretical interpretation of the relationship of aging to symbolism and ritual.

After a brief introduction to the connective and integrative functions of ritual, the functions, characteristics, and stages (separation, liminality, and reaggregation) of rites of passage are described. She notes that although life sequences seem to be segmented in all societies and recognized in large part through ritual, rituals marking early life stages and mortuary ritual are most evident while rituals marking transitions during the adult years are relatively sparse.

Other important aspects of ritual discussed include topics such as the human drive for reflexive knowledge and its relation to ritual, ritualized reminiscence, and the power of ritual to alter the emotional states of its participants and transcend time. Although most of the examples and discussion deal with public ritual and its individual and societal implications, some references to family ritual among the elderly are also made. These may be of particular interest to scholars who do not share the author's apparent tendency to understand ritual only as events of "high stylization" clearly distinguishable "from ordinary affairs."

6-14. Ragucci, A.T. (1990). The ethnographic approach and nursing research. In P.J. Brink (ed.), Transcultural nursing: A book of readings (pp. 163-174). Prospect Heights, Ill.: Waveland Press, Inc. Reprinted from A.T. Ragucci (1972). The ethnographic approach and nursing research. Nursing Research, 21(6), 485-90.

This reprint of an article first published in 1972 describes the method of participant observation utilized by the author in her unpublished Ph.D. dissertation on cultural continuity and change in the concepts of health, curing practices, and ritual expressions among Italian-American women. Several aspects of ethnographic methodology are discussed, including ethnoscience, the use of small groups, informal interviews, unobtrusive observation at diverse social occasions, and the importance of defining the researcher's role within the community studied in such a way as to facilitate his or her acceptance by them.

Exposure to her emphasis upon intracultural variations in health beliefs and practices could be of benefit to many ethnographic researchers since, as she points out, some studies disregard differences between generations and do not sufficiently take into account the first or immigrant generation. Of particular interest to the nurse contemplating ethnographic research are her discussion of the advantages and appropriate use of ethnography in nursing research, and her acknowledgement of the conflicts that may arise between the therapeutic and investigative roles of the nurse researcher when harmful activities are noted.

6-15. Ross, J.K. (1977). Socialization into the community. In J.K. Ross, Old people, new lives (pp. 106-125). Chicago: The University of Chicago Press.

Jennie-Keith Ross (who later uses the name of Jennie Keith) investigated community creation in a French retirement residence by living in the residence for a year as a participant observer. The process of socialization of new residents into the community is described in Chapter Six of the book. This chapter presents details regarding the organized arrival rituals which take place during the new residents' first day, the newcomers' entrance into the dining room and into formal organized activities, their development of informal ties, and the apparent influence of their pre-admission situations upon their present acceptance and behavior. Although the intent of the author was not specifically to investigate ritual behaviors, the ethnographic methodology which was utilized in this study provided rich enough data to enable a few rituals to be described in the chapter. Of greater interest is the possible interpretation that here is being described a rite of passage, even an extended initiation rite into a separate society. Reading this chapter can thus provided scholars in ritual studies with insights helpful for planning research and making comparisons with new residents in other types of elderly communities and institutions.

7

SLEEP AND AGING

Sarah B. Lamm

INTRODUCTION

"No small art it is to sleep. It is necessary for that purpose to remain awake all day." Nietzsche

Sleep-- nothing in our lives is more intimately related to our health and well being yet so often taken for granted. Human beings spend over one-third of their lives sleeping but physicians rarely include questions about sleep quality or quantity in patient examinations. Changes in the age distribution demographics of the United States will soon place an increased burden on an already strained health care economy.

Changes in quality and quantity of sleep are not necessarily inevitable consequences of the aging process, as once believed. While researchers continue to unravel the mystery of primary vs. secondary aging of the human body, some important facts regarding sleep and health have become quite clear.

The sleep wake cycle is one of many circadian rhythms. It is a biologically and environmentally driven process that completes itself within a 24 hour period in normal adult human beings. The regulation of sleep onset appears to be controlled by the brain stem. In order to accurately and efficiently study sleep, researchers and clinicians use polygraphic recordings of brain activity (EEG), muscle tone (EMG), heart rate (ECG) and respiration. With these measures, sleep can be broken into five stages and three main subtypes. Rapid eye movement (REM) sleep is characterized by high electrical activity in the brain, muscle atonia and distinctive bursts of eye movement. REM sleep is often associated with dreaming. Non-REM sleep is characterized by decreased electrical activity, variable muscle tone and changing awareness of internal and external stimuli. One specific kind of non-REM sleep is slow wave sleep

(SWS). SWS is sometimes called deep or quiet sleep. Brain activity slows and awareness of stimuli is diminished.

Sleep architecture is a way of describing the amount of each type of sleep and the pattern in which this sleep is achieved. Changes in sleep variables and architecture can signal sleep disorder or other changes in the body's homeostasis.

One of the most frequently diagnosed sleep disorders is sleep apnea, sometimes called sleep disordered breathing (SDB). Sleep apnea is the cessation of breath while sleeping. A small amount of sleep apnea is present in infants and the tendency to develop apnea increases with age and some medical conditions. There are two main types of sleep apnea. Obstructive sleep apnea occurs when the airway becomes occluded during sleep due to decreased muscle tone around the airway. Thoracic muscles continue to operate and eventually force air through the closed airway. Snoring and gasping are the result of sleep apnea. Central apnea results from a decrease of stimulation to the thoracic muscles from the brain. The airway remains open but the chest ceases to move for a period of time. More than five apneas per hour of night sleep is currently considered clinically significant. With each apnea the level of oxygen in the blood drops and level of carbon dioxide increases. In addition most apneas are accompanied by brief arousals. The immediate sequela of apnea are morning headache and drowsiness due to frequent arousals. The long term effects of sleep apnea include increased risk of stroke and cardiovascular strain. Current treatments for sleep apnea include uvulopalatopharyngioplasty, tracheostomy (surgeries to open the airway) and continuous positive airway pressure (CPAP). CPAP is applied through a nasal mask. An occluded airway is held open by positive pressure being forced through the airway.

Disorders of the sleep-wake cycle can be brought on or exacerbated by a variety of psychosocial and physiological processes that may accompany aging. Changes in social patterns with retirement, death of a spouse or loved one, and the depression that may follow these events can lead to severe disruptions of sleep. Concurrent disease states, cognitive changes with some neurodegenerative processes and medication to treat these diseases can also disrupt an already delicate circadian cycle.

With the obvious complexity of the aging human body, it is difficult to separate "normal" changes in sleep patterns due to aging from those associated with a more pathological origin. But, the fact remains that at least one half of those over the age of 65 who live independently in this country, and about two thirds of those in long term care facilities suffer from some disturbance of sleep. It is important to remember that disorders of the sleep-wake cycle affect not only the person with disturbed sleep but family, staff and caregivers as well.

The field of Sleep Disorders Medicine is rapidly acquiring literature in basic and clinical research that attempts to define "normal" sleep more clearly, describe specific disorders and test the efficacy of current and future treatment for these disorders. What follows is a liberal sampling from a variety of fields of expertise including some excellent resources and some common sense guides to understanding and improving the quality and quantity of sleep at any age.

Traditionally sleep studies are performed in sleep laboratories. Many of the bibliographies that follow are examples of sleep lab evaluation and protocol (Berry, 1986; Naifeh, 1987; Aldrich, 1989). Other researchers prefer a more naturalistic approach and have studied sleep in home environments using ambulatory monitoring techniques (Ancoli-Israel, 1987; Jacobs, 1989). Some classic literature reviews have also been included (Dement, 1982; Shwartz, 1989; Ancoli-Israel, 1989).

A number of practical guides to sleep assessment and treatment are now available to clinicians. Included in the bibliographies are some excellent examples (Hoch, 1986; McGinty, 1987; Bonnet, 1989). Recently a number of popular articles have been published to help educate the general public. The American Medical Association's "Guide to Better Sleep" (1984) and Lipman's "Stop Your Husband From Snoring" (1990) are particularly good examples.

ANNOTATED BIBLIOGRAPHY

7-1.   Aber, R., & Webb, W.B. (1986). Effects of a limited nap on night sleep in older subjects. Psychology and Aging, 1, 300-302.

Most older adults experience increased night awakenings as a part of the normal aging sleep pattern. There has been evidence that an excessive number of these night wakenings can lead to day time sleepiness. One common recommendation to combat this problem is a nap. However, there is concern that a day time nap may disturb an already fragile sleep pattern. This study addresses this question. Unfortunately the limitations of this study far out way the information it yields.

The sample size of 16 is rather small and all of the subjects were healthy, working females between the ages of 50 and 60. This may not fit the current definition of "older," more likely "middle aged." Subjects served as their own controls and were polysomnographically recorded for four nights. They were given an opportunity to nap on days one and three. Nap time was limited to one hour within the normal work day. The results showed no change in frequency of night wakening on nap days.

The questions surrounding the effect of a nap on the sleep of "older" subjects remains unanswered in my opinion. A larger, more diverse sample is needed as well as a systematic manipulation of nap times and lengths. This is an important issue to be pursued, especially for those involved in geriatric care.

7-2.   Aldrich, M., Eiser, A., Lee, M., and Shipley, J.E. (1989). Effects of continuous positive airway pressure on phasic events of REM sleep in patients with obstructive sleep apnea. Sleep, 12, 413-419.

    In this well designed and carefully executed study, REM (rapid eye movement) rebound was assessed in patients using CPAP (continuous positive airway pressure) for the first time. Patients suffering from severe apnea during sleep often experience a reduction of REM sleep due to frequent arousals following apneas. Treatment with CPAP allows for continuous periods of sleep and thus increased REM episodes. This study was designed to better define the effects of acute CPAP treatment on REM sleep and REM density. Twenty-six subjects with a mean age of 47 years were recorded polysomnographically. Results showed an increase in both frequency and density of REM episodes upon the first night of CPAP use.
    This study is an excellent example of sleep laboratory methodology and protocol. A plethora of useful descriptions and definitions are given. The author's discussion includes a comparison of the effect of CPAP on REM rebound to the effects that are present with other available methods for treating severe sleep apnea.

7-3.   American Medical Association. (1984). Guide to Better Sleep, Random House, New York.

    The American Medical Association calls this book, a "Straight-talk, No-nonsense, guide to Better Sleep," and that it is. I recommend the whole book, to be browsed, absorbed and looked to again and again.
    Important and sometimes complex biological topics are addressed in a clear, informative and well documented manner. A chapter entitled "The Later Years" deals with the evolution of sleep over the life span and explains common complaints of older adults such as snoring, muscle twitches and nighttime awakenings. This chapter also includes tips for regulating an unreliable inner clock. For someone who has questions about sleep - academic or personal - I suggest beginning here.

7-4.   Ancoli-Israel, S. (1989). Epidemiology of sleep disorders. Clinics in Geriatric Medicine, 5, 347-361.

    This informative article focuses on the nature and prevalence of some specific sleep complaints and disorders in the elderly. This review includes an excellent history of the epidemiological work that has been done in sleep disorders to date. Apnea and periodic leg movement syndromes are discussed in detail and prevalence statistics are provided.

In particular, the sections mentioned above are well written and full of useful descriptions and definitions. Other issues that are addressed include sleep apnea and neurologic impairment, sleep in nursing home populations and sleep apnea and morbidity. This article provides an overview of the epidemiological history and current state of research on the disorders listed as well as an extensive and essential reference section.

7-5.   Ancoli-Israel, S., Kripke, D.F., and Mason, W. (1987). Characteristics of obstructive sleep apnea in the elderly: an interim report. Biological Psychiatry, 22, 741-750.

Sonia Ancoli-Israel is one of the most respected sleep researchers in the field and is the foremost authority in alternative recording technologies for sleep assessment. This report gives the interim data from a larger project using the modified Respitrace Medilog recorder, an ambulatory recording system. The purpose of this investigation was to compare independently living elderly individuals with obstructive and central sleep apnea.

Three-hundred fifty-eight subjects were studied in their homes. A detailed description of the methodology and protocol are given . The limitations of this kind of home monitoring procedure are discussed by the authors. Results are given with respect to prevalence, apnea sub-groups, weight, age and gender, snoring and depression.

The authors' conclusions state that sleep apnea is prevalent in the elderly and is often associated with increased day time napping and more disturbed night time sleep. Differences in subjective sleep history, complaints and medical history provided no basis for discrimination of apnea sub-groups, however.

This is a fine report and an excellent example of the usefulness of ambulatory recording devices in the home.

7-6.   Ancoli-Israel, S., Parker, L., Sinaee, R., Fell, R.L., and Kripke, D.F. (1989).   Sleep fragmentation in patients from a nursing home. Journal of Gerontology: Medical Sciences, 44, M18-M21.

This particular investigation was one of the first to systematically record the sleep of nursing home patients in their natural sleeping environment. An ambulatory monitoring procedure called the "wrist actigraph" was used to record 15 hours of activity from 200 nursing home residents. A study of this size and method is an heroic effort as well as a landmark in this type of field research.

The article contains a brief history of the research on the sleep of nursing home residents and a detailed methodology. Results show that patients spend an average of 6.5 hours out of bed and require this increase in time in bed over the day to obtain a total of approximately 8 hours of sleep. This 8 hours was distributed over the 15 hours of recorded time with nearly 50 per cent of the subjects sleeping some portion of each hour.

The limitations of using only 15 hours from the 24 hour day are recognized by the authors; readers should interpret the results accordingly. Caution is especially indicated with respect to the results given on night wakenings. There appears to be a bias in the data due to medications, apnea and staff behavior differences. None of these factors were controlled for in this study.

The authors conclude their report by providing suggestions on ways to improve the sleep of this population and encouraging further investigations of this type.

7-7.   Berry, D.T., Phillips, B.A., Cook, Y.R., Schmitt, F.A., Honeycut, N.A., Edwards, C.L., Lamb, D.G., Morgan, L.K., and Allen, R.S. (1989). Sleep-disordered breathing in healthy aged persons: one year follow-up of day time sequelae. Sleep, 12, 211-215.

Sleep Disordered Breathing (SDB) involves breathing disturbances such as apneas, hypopneas and oxygen desaturation during sleep. In overweight, snoring, middle-aged men, SDB has been linked to deterioration in day time functioning. This implicates SDB as a health risk continuum, at least for some populations. It is known that SDB is frequently present in the elderly but its clinical significance remains unclear. Previous reports comparing SDB with increased morbidity in the elderly have had mixed results.

This report examines the one year follow-up of 29 healthy older persons who were previously studied with polysomnography and day time evaluations. Several relationships were shown between the SDB indices taken at baseline and the measures of day time functioning taken one year later. This is of importance since previous studies have failed to link SDB with concurrently measured day time functioning. Cardiopulmonary variables such as elevated systolic blood pressure and irregular heart beats were shown at follow-up to be related to the earlier SDB indices.

The authors recognize the limitations of the study including the small sample size, brief follow-up period and the myriad of statistical tests used. Nonetheless, this is an important work.

7-8.   Berry, D.T., Webb, W.B., and Block, A.J. (1986). Sleep apnea syndrome: a critical review of the apnea index as a diagnostic criterion. Chest, Oct., 4, 529-531.

This paper addresses the question of the utility of the current criterion of 5+ apneic episodes per hour of sleep in diagnosing Sleep Apnea Syndrome (SAS) in the aged. SAS is defined and a description of the evolution of the current criterion is given. The authors describe the literature review that was conducted in sleep research from 1973- 1982. A study was assembled using the quantitative data available on otherwise healthy individuals with apnea.

Results of this analysis showed that the false positive rate (apnea index >5 in normal subjects) is low in young healthy subjects. False positives were increased in those 60 years of age or older. A chi-square test was performed on another sample to assess the independence of age and a diagnostically significant level of apnea. A positive relationship was shown between age and the level of apneic activity. The authors conclude that the current standard criterion may not be appropriate in an elderly population. A number of studies have shown that an apnea index of 5+ does not predict an increase in health risk factors associated with SAS.

The authors give a possible explanation for the apparent misuse of the 5+ criterion: there were no subjects over the age of 60 in the original validation study that determined 5 as the cut-off. It is evident that more research is required to solve one of the longest standing debates in the sleep literature.

7-9.   Bliwise, D., Carskadon, M., Carey, E., and Dement, W. (1984). Longitudinal development of sleep-related respiratory disturbance in adult humans. Journal of Gerontology, 39, 290-293.

A number of cross-sectional studies have shown an increased prevalence of Sleep-Related Respiratory Disturbance (SRRD) with advancing age. This report provides a longitudinal analysis of SRRD and some other physiological measures related to breathing and sleep.

Fifteen elderly subjects were re-evaluated 2.8 years after their initial polysomnographic recording. The average age of the subjects was 73.6 at the time of follow-up. Ten middle-aged subjects were also re-evaluated approximately 8.1 years after their initial polysomnographic recordings. All subject were chosen because they showed a low SRRD index on their initial recording, were healthy and had no sleep complaints. Results showed no sex differences on either occasion. The SRRD index increased significantly from time 1 to time 2 for both groups. The authors present a detailed analysis of these results but caution against interpretation because of the limited sample size and follow-up period.

Issues of importance that are discussed include the need for longitudinal analysis of this kind, the effect of even modest weight gain on SRRD and the >5 respiratory disturbance index for determining Sleep Apnea Syndrome. This is an important and well designed study.

7-10. Blois, R., Feinberg, I., Gaillard, J.M., Kupfer, P.J., and Webb, W.B. (1983). Sleep in normal and pathological aging. Experientia, 39, 551-558.

This report begins with an interesting cross-sectional study of subjects between the ages of 20 and 60 years. Subjects were divided into four age groups (20-29, 30-39, etc.) and recorded in a sleep laboratory for three consecutive nights. Subjects were compared on all of the classic sleep parameters.

Sleep time was longer in the 20-29 year old group and decreased with age. Waking and stage 2 sleep also showed an age related decrease. REM (rapid eye movement) sleep remained proportionately stable across groups. Latency for stages 1, 2, 3 and REM sleep remained stable across groups as well. While stage 4 sleep could not be reliably measured, the authors note that several of the subjects in the older group had no stage 4 sleep at all. Sleep efficiency (a ratio of total sleep over time in bed) and sleep organization both decreased in the older groups.

The authors next present the results of an additional study concerning EEG (electroencephalography) wave form profiles in NREM (non-REM) sleep in young and elderly subjects. Finally, the issue of depression and aging is discussed and the results of a related study are shown. This study compared the EEG of elderly subjects with major depressive disorder syndrome and non-depressed elderly. There appears to be an age-related decrease in sleep efficiency, delta sleep and REM latency in elderly subjects with major depressive disorder.

This report is an interesting and exhaustive look at some major issues in sleep and aging. It is an ambitious work, albeit somewhat dated.

7-11. Bonnet, M.H., and Arand, D.L. (1989). Sleep loss in aging. Clinics in Geriatric Medicine, 5, 405-420.

This article begins with a brief discussion of sleep laboratory protocol, the effects of sleep loss in older persons and the use of hypnotic medications as a treatment for insomnia. The stages of sleep and classic characteristics of sleep used in analysis are described with respect to sleep loss and aging. In general, studies agree in describing the effects of sleep loss and recovery of sleep in this population. Slow wave sleep and REM (rapid eye movement) sleep show a rebound effect, and latency to sleep onset is increased with age.

A second part of this report focuses on changes in psychomotor performance during and after sleep loss. Recovery of baseline function is typically seen after one night of normal sleep, even following sleep loss of up to 64 hours. The implications of these results and the information provided from a study of chronic insomniacs are discussed.

This paper provides some detailed information on sleep deprivation and depression in older adults and has a solid theoretical framework.

7-12. Carskadon, M.A., and Dement, W.C. (1985). Sleep loss in elderly volunteers. Sleep, 8, 207-221.

These authors are both premier researchers in the area of sleep and aging. This study is a landmark in the field in that it was the first complete investigation of the effects of sleep deprivation on recovery sleep in a truly older age group. Previous studies have used subjects up to 50 years of age. The subjects described in this report are 10 volunteers aged 61-77 years, mean age 69.3. These subjects showed no intellectual deficits, dementia or psychiatric history. A description of the procedure is given. The authors note that none of the subjects had any difficulties with the sleep loss procedure, nor did they complain of any intolerable consequences of the sleep deprivation.

Nocturnal sleep on baseline night, recovery night 1 and recovery night 2 are described in great detail. Recovery sleep exhibited patterns similar to those shown in middle-aged subjects, but were somewhat short lived in the older subjects. Stage 4 sleep showed a continuous rebound response on recovery night 2. Performance, reported sleepiness and sleep latency appeared to recover more rapidly in the older subjects than was typically shown in the young.

The limitations of the current sleep parameter scoring criteria for the elderly are addressed. This report is a classic example of sleep laboratory investigation and protocol including a description of the one subject who would fit no analysis.

7-13. Dement, W.C., Miles, L.E., and Carskadon, M.A. (1982). "White paper" on sleep and aging. Journal of the American Gerontology Society, Jan., 30, 25-50.

This report was prepared by the top researchers in the field of sleep and aging and is based on a comprehensive review by the National Institute on Aging. This information was presented to the White House Conference on Aging. Its goal was to focus on the areas of sleep and aging that are most important for the well-being of older persons and future research.

Discussion is presented of survey literature. Several studies of merit are pointed out. The authors provide the definitive descriptions of the variables and sleep patterns derived from polysomnograms including sleep time, sleep latency, WASO (wake after sleep onset) and the sleep stages. Subjective complaints about sleep and daytime sleepiness are addressed along with the incidence and meaning of several specific sleep disorders present in the elderly. The report continues with a description of age-related changes in the sleep/wake cycle in humans and animals. Circadian and other biologic rhythms are included. The use of hypnotic medications in this population is also addressed. Finally, the recommendations of the White House Conference on Aging are given. This report is the definitive source for description, definition and references of related literature and is essential reading for anyone interested in the research of sleep and aging.

7-14. Haze, J.J., Govindan, S., Nahmias, J.S., and Fourre, J.A. (1987). Obstructive sleep apnea. Journal of Craniomandibular Practice, 5, 303-304.

This enlightening editorial provides a look at obstructive sleep apnea from a medical/surgical perspective. The authors refer to obstructive sleep apnea as "... not only a medical problem; (but) also a public health nightmare" due to the number of people in the country's work force who fall into a health risk category because of this disorder. This could include those who are obese, have hypertension or complain of chronic day time sleepiness. Caution is advised against the premature decision to try surgical procedures (neuromuscular craniomandibular principals) to treat obstructive sleep apnea given the current state of research on etiology and alternate therapies. Other methods of diagnosis and treatment are mentioned in an effort to advise those in surgical practice.

7-15. Hoch, C., and Reynolds, C. (1986). Sleep disturbances and what to do about them. Geriatric Nursing, 7, 24-27.

This article provides a basic but accurate look at sleep disturbance in the elderly. Written from a clinical point of view, and directed toward the practicing nurse, this paper describes symptomatically the changes in sleep that can occur with aging, illness, psychological impairment and medication. Sleep assessment by nursing professionals is encouraged. Some basic interventions are described that can be implemented if indicated. These interventions rely heavily on sleep hygiene therapy and are for use if medical attention is not immediately needed or available. Finally, polysomnographic evaluation is discussed and suggestions for its indication are given.

Nurses and care givers may find this article more to their liking than some of the other literature currently available. This report is accurate and easily applicable. Nurses and other care givers know their patients; they see them nap during the day and they must comfort them at night. This critical information about how a person is sleeping is often missed by the physician. For this reason, educated nurses can provide a sometimes urgent liaison between patient and sleep specialist.

7-16. Jacobs, D., Ancoli-Israel, S., Parker, L., and Kripke, D.F. (1989).

Twenty-four-hour sleep-wake patterns in a nursing home population. Psychology and Aging, 4, 352-356.

This study was designed to extend the findings of a report published earlier (Ancoli-Israel et al.,1989) using the wrist actigraph to monitor the 24 hour sleep/wake patterns of nursing home residents. Twenty subjects were selected from the same group that had been studied previously. All subjects completed the Dementia Rating Scale and the Geriatric Depression Scale.

The authors found subjects to sleep an average of 11.7 (SD 3.6) hours throughout the 24 hour recording period. Subjects slept approximately 40 minutes out of each hour in the sleep phase (6pm-8am) and as much as 32 minutes of the hour during the wake phase. Greatest amounts of wake were found in hours corresponding to meal times. The most intriguing finding to come from this study is the severe fragmentation of sleep in this population. None of the twenty subjects who were recorded had more than two consecutive hours of consolidated sleep.

The actigraph is worn about the wrist much like a wrist watch. A recording device is worn around the waist and a wire connects the actigraph to the recorder. Previous studies have shown this procedure to be a reliable indicator of some specific sleep/wake parameters in young and middle-aged persons. This procedure has not been validated against EEG (electroencephalography) in elderly under constant care. It is probable that this method of recording may have overestimated the inactivity of this population because of the sedentary nature of the subjects. The authors advise caution in interpreting the results. Despite its limitations, this is an important and methodologically respectable investigation.

7-17. Johnson, J.V. (1985). Drug treatment for sleep disturbances: Does it really work? Journal of Gerontological Nursing, 11, 8-12.

This clinical study was conducted to assess the nocturnal sleep patterns and the day time behaviors of older institutionalized adults. One group of subjects was already receiving hypnotics nightly. The Sleep Pattern and Daytime Behavior questionnaires were both used to quantify the subjects' sleep and waking patterns. Several conclusions are made by the author based on the information obtained from these surveys.

Some subjects perceived disruptions in sleep regardless of whether or not they had taken any medication before sleep. The majority of subjects in both groups had prolonged sleep latencies, frequent nocturnal wakenings and reported a lack of "deep sleep." The methods used in this study are practical for clinical research, but the validity of this kind of information is questionable. Self-report data on measures of sleep such as night wakenings and latency have been shown to be highly unreliable in the past.

The article concludes with suggestions for geriatric nurses that include recognizing the normal changes in sleep due to aging, identifying and eliminating the long term use of hypnotics and continuation of this type of clinical research.

7-18. Klink, M.E., Quan, S.F., and Webster, L. (1986). Sleep disorders in the elderly. Part 1 and Part 2. Drug Therapy, Mar., 16, 104-105.

This rather abbreviated look at sleep disorders in the elderly provides valuable information on therapies from a pharmacologist's point of view. The goal of the article is to demonstrate a practical approach for dealing with sleep problems in the elderly and to explore the guidelines for evaluating and treating sleep disorders.

In Part 1, a brief explanation of age related changes in sleep is provided. Unfortunately some of this information is now out-dated. Factors that may disrupt sleep are identified; these include drugs, environmental conditions, menopause and disease states. This section provides a nice quick reference chart of the effects of a number of drugs on sleep. Part 2 outlines some essential questions to be used to obtain a complete sleep history from a patient. Guidelines for referral to a sleep disorders clinic and currently available treatments for some disorders are discussed. The long-term use of hypnotics is clearly discouraged. The take home message from this report is clearly stated: treat the cause of the sleep disturbance, not the symptoms.

It is the opinion of most sleep professionals that all related disciplines must be educated in the area of sleep and sleep disturbances. The only effective approach to the treatment of sleep disorders is a multidisciplinary one. This article shows an inspirational step in that direction.

7-19. Knight, H., Millman, R.P., Gur, R.C., Sykin, A.J., Doherty, J.U., and Pack, A.I. (1987). Clinical significance of sleep apnea in the elderly. American Review of Respiratory Disorders, 136, 845-850.

This study was conducted to assess the validity of using the current criterion of 5+ respiratory events per hour with an elderly population. Elderly subjects frequently exceed this criterion. There is some question as to whether or not complications associated with high rates of apnea in younger subjects occur in older populations.

Twenty-seven subjects were studied on two consecutive nights. Daytime sleepiness, cognitive function and some cardiovascular parameters were assessed. Subjects were divided into two groups for analysis: those who had <5 events per hour and those who had >5 event per hour. These groups did not differ statistically with respect to age or weight.

The high apnea group was found to have a shorter latency to sleep onset and increased daytime sleepiness. This finding of increased sleepiness is a controversial one, and the authors qualify it. No differences were found between groups with respect to cardiac variables, hypertension or cognitive ability. It was concluded that the presence of more than 5 apneas per hour is not necessarily associated with significant clinical consequences in the elderly. This is an ongoing debate still being addressed by researchers. This study was well designed, researched and executed.

7-20. Lipman, D.S. (1990). Snore no more! Prevention, 42, 38-46.

"Snore No More" is an excerpt from Dr. Lipman's book entitled "Stop Your Husband From Snoring" (1990, Rodale Press). This article is obviously written for the lay-public, but it is an important one for that same reason.

Dr. Lipman has his facts straight and a good intention. However, his advice will raise some clinical eyebrows. Included in the article is a questionnaire to be completed by the snorer and his (or her) sleeping partner about the snorer's sleeping habits. This survey is a simple yet predictive screening device to identify those snorers who may have sleep apnea. It is true that the majority of those suffering from apnea are unaware of their disorder since the symptoms manifest themselves when the person is asleep. The apneic may only be aware of daytime sleepiness, a morning head-ache, frequent nighttime arousals or complaint from a partner. A list of self-help tips is provided. These tips may be of use in temporarily relieving the snoring of a partner, but are by no means intended as an alternative to medical evaluation.

This article may be of particular use if one knows a snorer and is concerned that this person may be apneic. More detailed, accurate information is available elsewhere, but this is the perfect article to leave "lying in plain sight".

7-21. Mason, W.J., Ancoli-Israel, S., and Kripke, D.F. (1989). Sleep apnea revisited: a longitudinal follow-up. Sleep, 12, 423-429.

Elderly subjects, ages 65 and older, who had been previously recorded using the modified Medilog Respitrace system were re-evaluated for this report. The purpose of the re-evaluation was to assess the stability of breathing disturbances and diagnostic rating indices. The mean duration between initial recording and follow-up was 4.6 years. Sleep periods were scored for total sleep time, WASO (wake after sleep onset), apneas and leg jerks.

No significant increases were found in the apnea index or the respiratory index over the four year follow-up. These results are compared to previous reports, qualified and discussed. The authors found an increase in the number of leg jerks among men over the follow up period suggesting that periodic leg movements may continue to increase beyond age 65.

This study is a well planned and carefully executed example of the efficacy of ambulatory monitoring procedures.

7-22. McGinty, D. (1987). Sleep disorders in the elderly: rationale for clinical awareness. Geriatrics, 42, 61-72.

In this article, Dr. McGinty presents an excellent case for including a sleep history in the primary care physicians' standard patient interview. He begins by dispelling the myth that all changes in sleep patterns occur simply as a natural function of aging and describes some of the symptoms that can be troublesome. Included in this paper are tables with valuable information on the most frequent diagnoses underlying sleep complaints in the elderly, cardiovascular disorders that accompany sleep apnea, and the signs that indicate a need for sleep evaluation. Readers will surely be surprised by the information contained in these lists. A diagram indicating anatomic changes in age-related sleep disorders is presented along with a detailed description of both occlusive (obstructive) and central apneas.

Finally, recommendations are given as to which symptoms should be quickly addressed and why sedative-hypnotic drugs should be avoided. This paper should be required reading for all general practitioners, elderly care professionals and anyone who is or will ever be over the age of 65.

7-23. Monk, T.H., and Moline, M.L. (1988). Removal of temporal constraints in the middle-aged and elderly: effects on sleep and sleepiness. Sleep, 11, 513-520.

This study is a classic example of circadian experimentation. Ten healthy middle-aged and elderly subjects were studied in two different environmental conditions. First, a four or six day "entrainment" period was conducted with each subject. All temporal cues were removed except for strict meal and bed times established in accordance with each subject's usual 24 hour routine. Subjects were subsequently released into a 12 to 26 day "free running" period with the subjects able to eat, sleep and rise whenever they felt it was appropriate. Both of these conditions are classic experimental procedures. The goals of the study were to determine if removal of temporal constraints would affect 1) subjective day/night cycle lengths, 2) sleep and time in bed, 3) sleep efficiency, 4) daytime subjective activation levels, and 5) slow wave sleep percentages. Both body temperature and blood samples were taken during polysomnography.

Subjective day lengths and temperature cycles were longer in the free running condition than in entrainment. Time in bed fractions were also greater in the free running condition, but actual sleep fractions were not increased. This reflects in a lower sleep efficiency. Alertness was greater in the free running condition, and peak alertness time came earlier.

The authors discuss the implications of these findings along with the issue of temperature cycle change as an explanation for the loss of sleep efficiency in the free running condition. Despite the small sample size, this is a wonderfully intensive and very interesting study that provides a glimpse into the human internal clock.

7-24. Naifeh, K.H., Severinghause, J.W., and Kamiya, J. (1987). Effect of aging on sleep-related changes in respiratory variables. Sleep, 10, 160-171.

This article examines several respiratory variables in 12 healthy older (60+ years) and 11 healthy younger (30-39 years) subjects during all night sleep recordings. The purpose of the study was to determine the effect of age on breathing during sleep. Subjects slept four consecutive nights in a sleep laboratory; night 1 data were discarded. Variables measured were apneas, hypopneas, standard sleep parameters, oxygen saturation, transcutaneous PcO_2 and estimated tidal volume.

Results showed significant differences between groups on standard sleep parameters, as was to be expected from previous reports. Differences were also shown between groups with respect to respiratory disturbance. There was an increase in number of arousals associated with respiratory disturbance in the older subjects. Oxygen saturation was lower in the older subjects than the younger subjects during wake and sleep.

The authors concluded that aging by itself does not affect sleep related changes in oxygen saturation, or PcO_2, although the increased incidence of respiratory disturbance does produce transient swings in these variables. This is an interesting study but it has a few methodological drawbacks. A small sample size indicates caution should be used when interpreting the results. One must also be careful when dealing with cross-sectional studies, not to over generalize in projecting results. A longitudinal study is indicated to fully assess the effects of increasing age on respiratory variables.

7-25. Orr, W.C., Altshuler, K.Z., and Stahl, M.L. (1982). Managing Sleep Complaints. Chicago: Year Book Medical Publishers, Inc.

This book provides a handy desk reference for practicing professionals to help with differential diagnosis of sleep disorders. Specific information on any disorder can be found along with identification of symptoms and possible therapies and treatments. Other sections include information on interaction of medical and psychiatric disorders and sleep as well as an extensive review of medications, tolerance and withdrawal effects.

The authors provide an evolution of clinical approaches to sleep therapy and an outline of the official diagnostic classifications of sleep disorders. A sample questionnaire is provided to aid those who require a detailed sleep history from their patients. The appendix of the book lists the names and addresses of all of the certified sleep disorders clinics in the United States and abroad.

This book is slightly outdated, but to my knowledge no other publication like it exists. It is the most complete clinical diagnostic tool available to the public and is an excellent resource.

7-26. Oswald, I. (1986). Drugs for poor sleepers? British Medical Journal, 292, 715.

This British editorial provides a few words from a viewpoint that is opposed to that of most sleep researchers. Dr. Oswald feels that benzodiazepine hypnotics are safe and effective and should be available over-the-counter to consenting adults. The doctor has a sarcastic and vaguely amused opinion of the non-pharmacologic therapies that are available for those with complaints of insomnia. No mention is made of the treatment of older individuals or over medication.

This paper is important reading. It helps describe and explain the current beliefs about hypnotic drug administration by physicians. Researchers and sleep professionals must be aware of the biases that exist in the medical world in order to be able to combat them.

7-27. Penzel, T., Amend, G., Meinzer, K., Peter, J.H., and von Wichert, P. (1990). MESAM: a heart rate and snoring recorder for detection of obstructive sleep apnea. Sleep, 13, 175-182.

The authors present a technical report on an ambulatory device designed to detect heart rate and breathing sounds at 1 sample per second. MESAM (Madus Electronics Sleep Apnea Monitor) was developed in West Germany and is intended for screening persons suspected of having sleep related breathing disorders, including apnea.

A growing body of literature involves the use of these "alternative technologies" that can be used to help preselect individuals who may be in need of a full sleep laboratory work up. A detailed description of the MESAM device and its protocol is given along with instructions for data processing and scoring procedures. This is an important paper emphasizing the need for and applicability of ambulatory monitoring devices. The reference section includes other essential reports that discuss alternative technologies.

7-28. Schirmer, M.S. (1983). When sleep won't come. Journal of Gerontological Nursing, 9, 16-21.

This report is a descriptive and easy to read guide for nursing professionals and it provides a great deal of useful clinical information. The author begins by discussing the physiology of sleep and he describes a few of the better known biological rhythms such as temperature and corticosteroids. The sleep stages are identified and described in relation to normal aging sleep patterns. An interesting but somewhat outdated discussion of the function of sleep is also included.

The article becomes clinically useful in its description of some common causes of sleep disruption. Physical illness such as thyroid imbalance, nocturnal angina, and hypertension can all cause sleeping abnormalities. Medications and lifestyles can also play a role in how efficiently a person sleeps. Guidelines are given for assessing sleep disorders in patients. Also provided in this discussion is an impressive strategy for obtaining a complete sleep history.

The implications of patients with sleep disorders for health care professionals are discussed. The author suggests some basic sleep hygiene as well as the appropriate administration of medication. For instance, patients with pain should be given their analgesics one-half hour before going to bed.

This article is easy to read, precise and to the point. I think it would be of great value to health care professionals. Nurses especially will benefit from this report if they have little or no background in sleep disorders.

7-29. Schwartz, A.R., and Smith, P.L. (1989). Sleep apnea in the elderly. Clinics In Geriatric Medicine, 5, 315-329.

The purpose of this report was to review the literature on sleep apnea with a focus on epidemiology. There is also an emphasis on recognition of the disorder by its symptoms and polysomnography, and how individual disorders relate to aging. The authors begin by defining and describing sleep apnea and distinguishing between central, obstructive and mixed apneas. Prevalence rates are discussed with respect to apnea in the elderly; a figure of 24 per cent is given. While age appears to be a factor in predicting apnea, obesity seems to be more highly related. One theory of the pathogenesis of sleep apnea is discussed in detail. The authors present evidence that a disruption in neural ventilatory regulation may be the most precise explanation for the disorder, at least in the elderly. Data from cardiac patients fit well into this theory.

Also included in this report is a large and very useful description of the clinical features of apnea. Symptoms such as snoring, choking, daytime somnolence and fatigue are discussed. Snoring and obstructive apnea have been associated with an increased incidence of hypertension, cerebrovascular disease, coronary artery disease and cardiac arrhythmias. There are conflicting reports, however, as to whether or not increased morbidity can be linked directly to apnea.

Clinical evaluation procedures as well as theories that are currently available are discussed. This is a detailed and accurate report on the status of the literature on sleep apnea and its effect on the elderly. I recommend this article for its information and resources.

7-30. Stone, W.S. (1989). Sleep and aging in animals: relationships with circadian rhythms and memory. Clinics In Geriatric Medicine, 5, 363-379.

This report is the most current review of the existing literature on sleep in aging animals. Part one discusses the methodological shortcomings of the past research on the sleep of laboratory animals. Recent studies have shown improvement and the results appear to be species differentiated.

Rats tend to sleep a little less as they age and their sleep gradually becomes more fragmented. Some strains show slightly different effects and these results are discussed. The literature on the effect of aging on sleep in mice is scarce and methodologically complicated. It appears that circadian amplitudes of waking, non-paradoxical sleep and paradoxical sleep are reduced in older mice. The research on cats shows an age x sex effect on reduction of some sleep states. These reductions in slow wave sleep, sleep bout length and the apparent fragmentation of sleep in older animals mimic the effects that older humans have. The relationships are discussed in detail. These relationships between sleep and other physiologic functions is addressed but the author notes that experimentation is scarce and no conclusions can be made.

The final section of this report deals with the interactions between sleep and cognitive functions. A current hypothesis that age related changes on sleep may be related to memory in old animals is discussed and evidence is presented to support this theory. For instance, some pharmacologic treatments used to enhance memory can also enhance sleep.

The author concludes with a status report of the literature available on animal sleep and aging. More research and publishing of detailed methodologies is needed to facilitate future reviews and meta-analyses. This is a fascinating report that contains a wealth of good information. The reference section is complete and useful.

7-31. Susman, J.L. (1989). Sleep in the elderly: a practical approach. Journal of Family Practice, 29 528-533.

In this report, the author provides readers with an informative and practical clinical guide to evaluating and treating sleep disorders in the elderly. A brief background on the physiology and purpose of sleep is included and a detailed guideline to the evaluation of sleep disorders is given. The most important things to consider in this process are obtaining a thorough sleep history, ruling out treatable underlying medical causes, elimination of drug and alcohol complications and knowledge of the normal aging sleep patterns.

The Association of Sleep Disorders Clinics has developed a classification system for the major sleep disorders. They include 1) disorders of the sleep/wake cycle, 2) disorders of excessive somnolence (DOES), 3) disorders of initiating and maintaining sleep (DIMS), and 4) other disorders. Each category is described and discussed in detail. Topics in the "other" category include narcolepsy, parasomnias, and the association of dementia to sleep. The author includes a list of good sleep hygiene tips for the elderly. Sleep hygiene is quickly becoming a preferred first line treatment for some people with disturbed sleep.

The final section of the paper deals with the currently available therapies for disordered sleep. Pharmacologic treatments are discussed. An interesting description of L-tryptophan is provided; however, since the publication of this article, L-tryptophan has been removed from the market because of adverse side effects. A flow-chart showing the metabolic rates of a number of commonly prescribed benzodiazepine hypnotics is given along with a very good discussion of their indications and contra-indications.

This article is an excellent resource and reference guide to the treatment of sleep disorders in the elderly. It is encouraging to see family physicians taking an active and informed role in the diagnosis and referral of those patients with troubled sleep.

7-32. White, D.P. (1988). Disorders of breathing during sleep: introduction, epidemiology and incidence. Seminars In Respiratory Medicine, 9, 529-533.

Dr. White provides an easy to read paper that helps define and explain disorders of breathing during sleep. His introduction reviews the sleep stages and the respiratory uniqueness of each as well as defining some commonly misinterpreted words such as apnea, hypopnea and respiratory events index. A description is given of arterial oxygenation during sleep as well as the normal or asymptomatic respiration that can occur. A good argument is presented for not basing therapy solely on the number of apneas recorded per night.

The sections on epidemiology and incidence are rather vague and offer nothing beyond the current basic knowledge of the profession. For a more in depth discussion of epidemiology or incidence one should look elsewhere.

8

HYPNOTIC DRUG USE AMONG THE ELDERLY

Sarah B. Lamm

INTRODUCTION

It is now understood that sleep changes as a function of normal aging. Research has shown that the duration and frequency of sleep episodes as well as the composition of the sleep state itself may be altered by increasing age. While the exact nature of these changes has yet to be precisely described, most elders and their health care providers are well aware of the effects of disorders of the sleep-wake cycle.

It has been estimated that 90% of those 60 to 80 years of age have had complaints of insomnia at one time. These complaints may be brought about by a change in lifestyle, loss of a spouse or other loved one, multiple disease states that may occur with age or a myriad of other psycho-social factors, including misinformation about what "normal" sleep actually is.

Historically, the most common method of addressing a complaint of insomnia has been the prescription of a "sleeping pill." Many medications can be used to induce drowsiness. The most widely prescribed somnolant is the sedative-hypnotic. In 1985 James reported that 35% of all independently living elders surveyed and 34% of those in skilled nursing facilities used hypnotics regularly. More recently investigators have reported that the prevalence of hypnotic drug use among the elderly remains high, and tends to change with age, gender and intensity of care within institutions. In several countries increases have been shown in overall drug use with increasing age. Hypnotic medications are primarily responsible for these increases. Exact prevalence rates are difficult to determine due to the classification of hypnotics with other psychotropic drugs in many studies. It is clear that hypnotic use among the elderly remains high despite the dangers involved with the chronic use of such drugs. Hypnotics can be especially threatening to older adults with respect to compound, dose, duration and polypharmacological interactions.

Advances in the diagnosis and treatment of sleep disorders have given physicians many options for the treatment of insomnia. Short term use of hypnotics when accompanied by behavioral interventions and close monitoring can be beneficial for most people who suffer from insomnia. The danger remains in chronic, unsupervised use of hypnotics in older patients. Current trends show a movement toward shorter acting drugs, lower doses and an increase in the use of anti-depressants to aid sleep in some patients.

The following articles are historical contributions in the continuing project of assessing the prevalence of the use of sedative hypnotics among the elderly and the effects of use. Some researches have attempted to asses the prevalence of hypnotic use among the elderly by conducting surveys in hospitals or long-term care facilities (Salsman, 1980; Morgan, 1981, 1982, and 1988). Controlled studies of the effect of certain hypnotics on overnight sleep architecture and daytime performance have also contributed to the field (Kales, 1974 and Nagel, 1978). Many papers have been published to aid clinicians in understanding hypnotics and to assist them in prescribing these drugs (Thompson, 1983; Reynolds, 1985 and Roehrs, 1989).

ANNOTATED BIBLIOGRAPHY

8-1. Bayer, A.J., and Pathy, M.S. (1985). Requests for hypnotic drugs and placebo response in elderly hospital inpatients. <u>Postgraduate Medical Journal</u>, <u>61</u>, 317-320.

In this report, the investigators established a placebo response in patients who would normally have taken an hypnotic to induce sleep. Out of 390 elderly patients requesting sleeping pills in the target hospital, 216 were completely satisfied with their sleep while taking a placebo throughout their hospital stay. A detailed description of the procedures and results is given. The authors claim that most of the hypnotics prescribed to elderly patients are unnecessary and tend to be for staff convenience. Assessment of satisfaction with sleep is, after all, a very subjective matter.

This article includes an exceptional introduction and conclusion to complement it's rather impressive results. The methodology of the study is sound and innovative.

8-2. Bruce, S.A. (1982). Regular prescribing in a residential home for elderly women. <u>British Medical Journal</u>, <u>284</u>, 1253-1257.

This rather informal report comments on one researcher's attempt to review and revise current drug regimens of 20 elderly group home residents. The focus of the study was to minimize drug interactions while maximizing cost effectiveness by eliminating unneeded drugs.

This is not a particularly interesting or skilled study but it does bear witness to an alarming fact. The investigator goes to great pains to withdraw patients from drugs deemed "no longer necessary" yet he says, "Hypnotics are also very difficult to withdrawal, particularly since patients are put to bed rather early in the evening." This shows a serious lack of education, as well as an intolerance of the normal changes in sleep patterns that accompany aging.

8-3. Christopher, L.J., Ballinger, B.R., Shepherd, A.M., Ramsay, A., and Crooks, G. (1978). Drug prescribing patterns in the elderly: a cross-sectional study of in-patients. Age and Aging, 7, 74-82.

A one day cross-sectional survey was conducted in July 1975, to assess the frequency of drug prescription in elderly inpatients. A total of 873 patients were surveyed then classified by patient category and drug group. Details of procedures and results are provided. The average number of drugs prescribed per patient was 3.3. Prevalence rates for hypnotic use ranged from 40 per cent to 70 per cent depending on the ward. Specific problems that were highlighted include no dose reduction with increasing age and multiple drug administration within a pharmacological group. Doses and dose schedules inconsistent with manufacturer's guidelines for the aged were found. A discussion of solutions is presented by the authors; for instance, decreasing dose of benzodiazepines with age and utilizing more effective scheduling for administration of hypnotics.

This is an informative and methodologically sound investigation. Reference is made to a possible reason for such high use of hypnotics in the sample obtained: low patient to physician ratio, that is, convenience.

8-4. Ingman, S.R., Lawson, J.R., Pierpaoli, P.G., and Blake, P. (1975). A survey of the prescribing and administration of drugs in a long-term care institution for the elderly. Journal of the American Gerontological Society, 7, 309-316.

This report was prepared as a part of a larger project on patterns of care in an extended care facility. The authors conducted a survey on the prescription and administration of drugs paying particular attention to those medications of the neuroactive class.

The number of drugs prescribed per patient differed from the number actually administered because of the large number of "as needed" prescriptions. Hypnotics were the third most commonly prescribed drugs with a prevalence rate of 23 per cent. Physicians were subsequently ordered to rewrite patient drug orders every thirty days. A follow up survey showed a decline in the number of drugs prescribed.

Recommendations for strict surveillance of drug regimens and some organizational changes are given by the authors. This paper is an important one in that it outlines specific changes that needed to be made in practice. This influential report was published in 1975 and today thirty-day review of drug lists is a relatively standard practice.

8-5. James, D. (1985). Survey of hypnotic drug use in nursing homes. Journal of the American Gerontological Society, 33, 436-439.

A survey of patients was conducted within two intermediate-care facilities and three skilled nursing facilities. Ten per cent of the patients polled received an hypnotic regularly or "as needed." This figure is lower than most previously reported rates. This could be due in part to the volunteer bias of the sample.

The three most commonly prescribed hypnotics were shown to have been administered for absurdly long times, from 11 weeks (triazolam) to 82 weeks (flurazepam). Given that most hypnotics have only been shown to be effective at inducing sleepiness for approximately 14 days, these extended durations are somewhat alarming. It was also shown that there was little, if any, dose reduction with age as is recommended by most hypnotic drug sheets.

The authors compare this study to previous reports and discuss the possible hazards of high dose/prolonged use of hypnotic medications in the elderly. This study is informative and well referenced, albeit slightly flawed methodologically.

8-6. Kales, A., Bixler, E.O., Tan, T., Scharf, M.B., and Kales, J.D. (1974). Chronic hypnotic-drug use: ineffectiveness, drug withdrawal insomnia, and dependence. Journal of the American Medical Association, 277, 513-517.

In this report, the authors address the problem of chronic hypnotic use in a systematic, experimental fashion. Insomniac patients who had been using hypnotics chronically for periods ranging from months to years were monitored in a sleep laboratory. These patients were then compared to chronic insomniacs who had received no drugs.

The results show a change in REM (rapid eye movement) sleep in the chronic hypnotic group with respect to the frequency and number of episodes as well as a delay in REM onset. Stage 4 sleep was decreased or eliminated altogether in chronic hypnotic users, depending on age. Overall, the younger insomniac patients using medication had higher wake time values (less sleep) than did the non-drug insomniacs.

While it appears that chronic hypnotic use will only worsen the insomniac condition, abrupt withdrawal is not suggested by the authors. The clinical implications of these findings are given through a case report.

8-7. Kripke, D.F., Simons, R.N., Lawrence Grafinkle, M.A., and Hammond, E.C. (1979). Short and long sleep and sleeping pills: is mortality increased? Archives of General Psychiatry, 36, 103-116.

This report focuses on the available epidemiologic data and the clinical issues surrounding the use of "sleeping pills" in lieu of controlled experimental data, which is limited. Hammond's "too much, too little" report from 1964 stated that too little sleep (less than six hours) or too much sleep (more than nine hours) may be associated with increased mortality. This matter is addressed along with more recent information that clarifies his original assertions that linked increased morbidity to the length of night sleep.

The data used to prepare this article were obtained from questionnaires used by the American Cancer Society. These questionnaires were not originally intended to assess sleep habits; the methodology is discussed and qualified. Data on self-reported sleep histories and subsequent mortality are provided.

This report is an interesting look at the sleep habits of a large, widely distributed sample. The authors conclude that unusually long or short sleep durations as well as the use of "sleeping pills" can be useful mortality risk predictors.

8-8. Morgan, K. (1983). Sedative-hypnotic drug use and ageing: a review. Archives of Gerontology and Geriatrics, 2, 181-199.

This informative review addresses the subject of hypnotic use in the elderly with respect to four categories of information: prevalence, type and dose, duration, and frequency of use. The authors conclude that prevalence rates for hypnotic use have remained high between 1960 and 1982, especially within institutions. Temporal trends and sex differences in use are explained. The authors find no consistent approach to minimizing the dangers involved in high dose, long duration or drug interaction with hypnotic medications.

This is the definitive review to date on this topic. It is easy to read, full of information and the references are of course, extensive. I consider this essential reading.

8-9. Morgan, K., Dallosso, H., Ebrahim, S., Arie, T., and Fentem, P. H. (1988). Prevalence, frequency, and duration of hypnotic drug use among the elderly living at home.   British Medical Journal (Clinical Research), 296, 601-602.

      Data taken from an activity and aging survey used for another project showed a prevalence rate of 16 per cent for hypnotic use among elderly living at home. Seventy-three per cent reported having taken hypnotic medications for at least one year and 25 per cent had durations of more than 10 years. It is widely known that the effectiveness of this type of medication is limited to approximately 14 days with the exception of flurazepam which can be of use for approximately 28 days.

      This study does much to examine this group of hypnotic users as well as some of the drugs being used. The report advises of the risks of prolonged hypnotic use and has a superb reference list.

8-10. Morgan, K., and Gilleard, C.J. (1981). Patterns of hypnotic prescribing and usage in residential homes for the elderly.   Neuropharmacology, 20, 1355-1356.

      A one day cross-sectional survey was conducted of all residents in local Authority homes (structured housing for the elderly) in one region of Scotland to determine patterns of hypnotic usage in residential homes for the elderly. A total of 33.5 per cent of the subjects polled took at least one hypnotic daily. A number of those on hypnotics were concurrently receiving other centrally acting drugs.   No preference was shown for the use of hypnotics with shorter half-lives.

      This study is methodologically sound and very informative. When combined with another study (Morgan, Gilleard, 1982), some longitudinal analyses are available.

8-11. Morgan, K., Gilleard, C., and Reive, A. (1982). Hypnotic usage in residential homes for the elderly: a prevalence and longitudinal analysis. Age Aging, 11, 229-234.

      In this report, Morgan et al. conducted a survey much like the one used in the previous year (Morgan, et al., 1981). The method of data acquisition was a one day cross sectional study of residents living independently in Authority homes in Scotland. The author reports that 34 per cent of the residents were using hypnotics and showed no preference for drugs with shorter half-lives. The most frequently prescribed hypnotic was nitrazepam, a particularly long acting drug associated with confusional states in the elderly. When compared to the previous study, little overall variation in prescribing patterns was shown. The report also points out the extended durations of hypnotic use among this population. Some words of explanation are given including patients' developing a preference to certain hypnotics and then resisting withdrawal or substitution.

The Morgan studies, viewed together, make up a valuable piece of the literature on hypnotic use in the elderly living independently.

8-12. Nayal, S., Castledon, C.M., George, C.F., and Marcer, D. (1978). The effect of an hypnotic with a short half-life on hangover effect in old patients. Age Aging, 7 (supplement), 50-54.

This paper describes a carefully planned and executed study of sedation, impairment of psychomotor performance, and EEG (electroencephalogram) abnormalities the morning after hypnotic use at bed time. Residual concentrations of circulating drug are responsible for these changes in function.

Appropriate amounts of two different drugs were administered at night on two occasions that were separated by at least three days. Twelve hours after the drug was taken, subjects were given a psychomotor test and a visual analog scale on which to rate their subjective levels of sleepiness. Results show a persistence of pharmacological action in the morning and a cumulative effect with both drugs tested.

The authors conclude that hypnotics have three specific side effects; hang-over, accumulation and dependence. Each effect is discussed with regards to the elderly.

8-13. Reynolds, C.F., Kupfner, D.J., Hoch, C.C., and Sewitch, D.E. (1985). Sleeping pills for the elderly: are they ever justified? Journal of Clinical Psychiatry, 46, 9-12.

This article examines, from a clinical perspective, the problems that can arise from sedating the elderly. Issues addressed include day time hang-over effect, impairment of function, drug interactions, drug tolerance and rebound insomnia. Etiologies of sleep disturbance in the elderly are discussed in detail with the use of some technical concepts. An in depth look at what the authors consider to be the "appropriate clinical assessment" is presented. This assessment includes patient history interview questions and explains the indications for polysomnography. A section on non-pharmacologic alternatives for the treatment of some disorders is presented. The report emphasizes education and further research.

Finally, the authors outline strict considerations for prescribing sedatives and benzodiazepine hypnotics for the elderly. This is an informative and well researched paper; for clinicians this is essential reading.

8-14. Roehrs, T.A., and Roth, T. (1989). Drugs, sleep disorders and aging. Clinics in Geriatric Medicine, 5, 395-403.

The authors provide a brief discussion of the changes in pharmacokinetics during normal aging and how these changes can complicate diagnosis and treatment of sleep disorders. An excellent report on depressant and stimulant use in aging is given including some recommendations for the use of such drugs.

Drug induced insomnia is discussed with explicit examples of common causes like the use of caffeine and other methylxanthines and depressants. Drug interactions with particular sleep pathologies such as sleep related breathing disturbances (apnea) and periodic leg movements are described.

This article is an excellent quick reference, but much more detailed descriptions of these topics are available elsewhere.

8-15. Salsman, C., and Van Der Kolk, B. (1980). Psychotropic drug prescriptions for elderly patients in a general hospital. Journal of the American Gerontological Society, 28, 18-22.

A one day cross-sectional survey was conducted in a Boston teaching hospital to assess the prevalence of the administration of centrally acting drugs. A lower age limit of 60 was set for inclusion. Doses were found to be more age appropriate than in some previous studies, but some drugs such as anti-depressants were often over prescribed.

This study has a complex design that breaks down the data into very descriptive groupings including a table of all the neuroleptic drugs used to treat patients with symptoms of confusion. This investigation found that nearly 75 per cent of the patients surveyed received hypnotics for the promotion of sleep. This is a relatively elevated number, even for an in-patient population.

This study is methodologically sound, albeit fairly complex. The specific details of neuroleptic drug prescription are informative and enlightening.

8-16. Thompson, T.L., Moran, M.G., and Nies, A.S. (1983). Psychotropic drug use in the elderly (part I). New England Journal of Medicine, 308, 134-138.

This report addresses the prescription patterns, demographic data and clinical considerations surrounding psychotropic drug use in the elderly. Changes in pharmacokinetics including absorption, distribution, and elimination are discussed. Screening procedures are suggested prior to the administration of drugs to treat sleep related symptoms in the elderly. A detailed and effective protocol is described and strongly recommended. Guidelines and precautions are also discussed for some drugs, particularly anxiolytics and hypnotics. The sleep stage alterations and current demographics are given for each type of drug.

This report is clinically relevant and should be required reading for all health care professionals, including practicing physicians.

9

ALZHEIMER'S DISEASE

Mary Ann Kistner

INTRODUCTION

One of the highest priority health issues associated with aging is Alzheimer's disease, a form of dementia. Dementia, a general term, is broadly defined as impairment of intellectual functioning of various causation. In contrast to multi-infarct dementia (MID) which occurs in persons with cardiovascular disease and is characterized by recurrent small strokes, or mixed dementia which is used to define either a combination of Alzheimer's disease and MID or dementias attributable to Parkinson's disease, advanced alcoholism, or other diseases causing cognitive impairment, Alzheimer's disease (AD) or dementia of the Alzheimer's type (DAT) is of unknown causation and is characterized by the presence of neurofibular tangles and by Alzheimer's plaques in the brain. Alzheimer's disease is thought to occur in about 50% of the cases of dementia and cannot be reliably diagnosed; confirmed diagnosis is only through autopsy. Additionally, there is not an effective treatment modality to either reverse or delay the effects of the disease. In the United States the cost of care for the estimated 4 million individuals with dementia amounts to more than 88 billion dollars annually.

This chapter provides an eclectic sampling of the literature of dementia, particularly of the Alzheimer's type, from the areas of biological, medical, psychological, and social research. Drawing from these many perspectives, the reader is exposed to the complex nature of the Alzheimer's "problem" and a feeling for the variety of foci that the research has assumed.

Four of the presented articles involve changes in physiological functioning which may be associated with Alzheimer's disease. These changes are being explored for their possibilities as diagnostic tools. Research studies of this kind have been conducted in hospitals or other clinical facilities where researchers have access to both probable Alzheimer's patients and a similarly matched control group. The study by Otsuka and others examines possible changes in Circadian patterns associated with blood pressure and heart rate in those with suspected Alzheimer's disease. Vitiello and associates monitor the sleep patterns of probable mildly affected AD patients while a study by Ship and others is concerned with determining possible differences which occur in salivary flow. Finally, a study by Husain and Nemeroff reviews the experimental literature regarding changes in neuropeptides that are associated with Alzheimer's disease and draws some conclusions regarding the feasibility of using changes in neuropeptide concentration to diagnose Alzheimer's disease.

The articles by Coyne and others, Folstein and associates, Mungas, Teri and Wagner, and Wade and others cite research concerned with both diagnosis and assessment of Alzheimer's disease in various settings. From the relatively uncomplicated use of the Mini-Mental Status Exam (MMSE) by physicians or other practitioners in an office setting, to the more complex clinical assessments done at diagnostic centers, the procedures followed are elaborated. Additionally, the implications of these diagnosis/assessment procedures and research outcomes are explored in some of these studies.

Three articles focus on cognitive deterioration associated with Alzheimer's disease. Fromholt and Larsen explore the patterns of deterioration of autobiographical memories over the life span. Cooper and others explore the association between cognitive deterioration and the expression of what are considered to be abnormal behaviors; this article also is concerned with assessment of abnormal behaviors associated with Alzheimer's disease. The final article in this group by Flint is an extensive literature review on the pathophysiology of delusions, hallucinations, and depression associated with Alzheimer's disease as well as the utility of using antipsychotic drugs in treatment.

An area in which there has been great interest has been the genetic transmission of Alzheimer's disease. There are strong implications of a relationship between early onset Alzheimer's disease and chromosome 21 and the genes located on that chromosome. Additionally, there may be the possibility of genetic involvement of other chromosomes in later onset Alzheimer's disease. Two articles, one by Heston and others and the other by Nalbantoglu and associates explore the family implications of Alzheimer's disease.

Finally, three articles are concerned in part or in whole with the impact of psychological and social factors and the expression of behaviors associated with Alzheimer's disease. The article by Kitwood addresses the dialectics of dementia. Two other previously mentioned articles, the one by Cooper and associates and the other by Flint, implicate psychological and/or social factors associated with the expression of dementia in addition to the physiological factors. Of great concern by social scientists is the cycle of regression in cognition which occurs as self-confidence in cognitive ability is eroded. The deficiency is reinforced by family members who may contribute to making the individual feel less confident and competent which further erodes self-confidence. The cycle of loss continues.

Together these fifteen articles present an overview of the types of research which are broadly concerned with the diagnosis and assessment of Alzheimer's disease. The amount of research which is being undertaken and the literature being produced is significant. As is indicated by the abstracts, there is great diversity in this research.

ANNOTATED BIBLIOGRAPHY

9-1. Cooper, J.K., Mungas, D. & Weiler, P.G. (1990). Relation of cognitive status and abnormal behaviors in Alzheimer's disease. Journal of the American Geriatric Society, 38, 867-870.

The study reported information gathered on 680 subjects brought to California Alzheimer's Diagnostic and Treatment Centers to be evaluated for Alzheimer's disease. Personal histories, physical examinations, laboratory data, and data regarding abnormal behaviors observed by caregivers and persons performing the medical examination and the tests at the Center were collected. The behaviors noted were entered into a principal components analysis which loaded on six factors: anger/agitation, depression, delusions/hallucinations, wandering, personality change, and insomnia. The presence or absence of these behaviors, in conjunction with the Folstein Mini-Mental State Examination (MMSE) and age, gender, duration of dementia, race, and education for each of the subjects were tested in a logistic regression. Results indicated that all behaviors except depression increased with declining MMSE scores and degree of cognitive impairment; the relationship with depression was less clear. However, it must be noted that there is great variability between various patients; overall statistically significant associations were weak, indicating that the level of cognitive functioning plays only a small part in the prevalence of these behaviors and that other variables also are involved.

Overall, the methodology seemed appropriate. The results indicated that assessment based on cognitive function loss is not very successful in predicting behaviors. Less than 10% of the variability in behaviors is caused by decrease in cognitive functioning; almost none is associated with the other variables of age, race, and gender; and none is associated with education or duration of dementia. Even in cases of severe cognitive impairment, the percentage of individuals exhibiting a behavior exceeded 50% only in anger/agitation and personality change/apathy; all other behavioral expressions ranged from about

22% to less than 40%. Consequently, this method of prediction of behavior based on cognitive impairment is not useful for caregivers and others who work with those with probable diagnosis of Alzheimer's disease.

9-2. Coyne, A.C., Meade, H.M., Petrone, M.E., Meinert, L.A. & Joslin, B.L. (1990). The diagnosis of Dementia: Demographic characteristics. The Gerontologist, 30, 339-344.

Individuals are referred to the Comprehensive Services on Aging Institute for Alzheimer's Disease and Related Disorders in New Jersey for diagnostic services to determine the extent of their cognitive impairment. Extensive medical testing of the referred person and case history information from both the referred individual and accompanying family member/caregiver are evaluated by a team of various professionals. A diagnosis is made and a plan of care developed with recommendations for follow-up. Of the 242 clients seen during the time of the study, the results for 239 are presented in statistical detail, and a summary is also made based on three groups: dementia of Alzheimer's type, 89 cases; multi-infarct dementia, 79 cases; and other diagnoses, 71 cases. The Alzheimer's type dementia patients were significantly older than those with multi-infarct dementia (76.2 vs 73.0) and those with other diagnoses (70.2 years). There were diagnostic differences based on the sex of the client as well as differences in hospitalization rates for the different groups; multi-infarct dementia had the greatest hospitalization rate. This article makes several hypotheses regarding the high incidence of multi-infarct dementia in the group, the increased rates of hospitalization of multi-infarct dementia patients, and the relative lack of significant impairment of that group. In summary, the overall thrust of the study was to gather information regarding patients who were diagnosed with dementia type disorders.

This study is a compilation of data from the records of the clinic and presents interesting demographics of the members of the study and their diagnoses. However, none of the findings were adequately explained, providing only limited information for others who are also concerned with care of cognitively impaired family members.

9-3. Flint, A.J. Delusions, hallucinations and depression in Alzheimer's disease: A biological perspective. (1991). American Journal of Alzheimer's Care and Related Disorders & Research, 6, 21-28.

An extensive review of available literature on the pathophysiology associated with hallucinations, delusions, and depression in patients with Alzheimer's Disease (AD) is presented. Studies associated with both delusions and hallucinations from the areas of neuropsychology, sensory impairment, neuroradiology, and neuropathology are reviewed. The findings of these studies are often unclear and contradictory, but the author speculates and makes some tentative hypotheses regarding the discrepancies and their possible causes. Additionally, the relationship between depression and dementia is explored in studies from neuropsychology, neuroradiology, neuropathology, and genetics with hypotheses formed to illuminate discrepancies. Findings indicate that AD elders are at higher risk for depression than are non-demented elders. A comparison of the effects of antipsychotic drugs in the treatment of both hallucinations and delusions in AD patients is presented; hallucinations are less responsive to drug treatments than are delusions. In the few studies which used placebo controls, a placebo effect was found, indicating that factors other than drugs enter into the management of the psychosis associated with AD. These findings indicate only minimal support for the use of antipsychotic drugs to treat psychotic symptoms which complicate AD. In the case of depression, there was also improvement with both antidepressive drugs and placebos, indicating the importance of other factors such as psychosocial stimulation and psychotherapy in treatment.

The conclusions of the article regarding the etiology of symptomatology of delusions, hallucinations, and depression which influence AD are extremely speculative. However, the author highlights deficiencies in the studies and provides future directions for research. A discussion of the utilization of both pharmacological and physical treatments is also presented. The importance of better controls, particularly the importance of testing with placebos, is emphasized. In general, this is a very thorough review of the literature pertinent to the topic.

9-4. Folstein, M.F., Bassett, S.S., Anthony, J.C., Romanoski, A.J. & Nestadt, G.R. Dementia: Case ascertainment in a community survey. (1991). Journal of Gerontology, 46, M132-138.

This study is the third part of a multi-stage study to ascertain the prevalence of dementia in an Eastern Baltimore community based sample. The focus of this particular article is to present expanded prevalence rates, to elaborate the procedures followed for ascertaining dementia, and to note methodological issues which may affect accurate case detection. The procedures followed for diagnosis and assignment to the particular dementia subgroups of multi-infarct dementia, Alzheimer disease, or mixed dementia, are carefully elaborated, and prevalence rates based on gender, race, and education for each of the three dementia sub-groups are presented. Findings indicated that males had slightly higher prevalence rates than females, and that there were differences in diagnosis as to type of dementia. Also, the more educated showed greater prevalence of dementia. Additionally, non-whites had prevalence rates almost twice as high as whites. Finally, as age increased, the prevalence of probable Alzheimer's disease, as well as multi-infarct dementia, increased. The authors compared their findings with several other studies using similar methodology and found comparable results.

The most significant problem with the overall study was the loss of participants over the course of the three stages. The total participating sample for stage three was 22 cases, only 40% of those eligible, and too few cases to allow for statistical comparison. Additionally, there may be confounding of age and education. Also, it may be questioned whether an East Baltimore sample is generalizable to the population as the authors suggest; this particular sample has a very low educational level and almost 50% is non-white. Whether the lack of variability in the sample is an effect of dementia or of sample attrition is not indicated in the study. However, without clarification, this would make the overall predictability rate to the non-institutionalized population suspect. On the positive side of this study is the definition and explanation of choice for inclusion in this sample. Additionally, the authors present readable tables to supplement the verbal presentation of the findings.

9-5. Fromholt, P. & Larsen, S. (1991). Autobiographical memory in normal aging and primary degenerative dementia (Dementia of Alzheimer type). Journal of Gerontology, 46, P85-P91.

This study compares reminiscent memory of a normal, non-demented elderly sample with three levels of demented adults who were matched for sociodemographics and overall health. The diagnosis of primary degenerative dementia (senile dementia of the Alzheimer's type or SDAT) was based on information from staff descriptions (50% of SDAT were institutionalized), patient journals, and information regarding the disease history. The findings were based on narrative interview data of most significant life events and a meta-memory questionnaire. The results indicated significant differences between the combined demented groups and the normal group regarding the number of words used, the number of memories recalled, the repetition of the same memories, the amount of detail presented, the number of non-episodic comments, the salience of transitional events, and the mix of positive, negative, and neutral events/emotionality. Although the pattern of memories was similar for the two groups, there were differences in distribution of memories across the life span and in the chronology of memory retrieval. Additionally, there were significant differences within the three demented groups on number of words used, number of memories recalled, and the amount of detail presented. Dementia was associated with both loss of memories and with loss of detail of those events which were remembered. Transitional events, those events important to the individual, were more preserved among the demented than were non-transitional events. Overall, as dementia progressed, it became increasingly difficult for subjects to maintain a coherent personal history.

This study provided memory pattern results which were considerably different from patterns obtained by the more commonly used prompt word method in which the most recalled events are recent. This study showed patterns of strong early memory, decreased memory of mid-life events, and increased recent memory. Several other studies using vivid memories have had similar findings. In general, this study was well-conceived, well-executed, and maintained sample controls. The methodology was carefully designed and the data clearly interpreted. A number of tables were included to summarize the findings, and these were particularly useful in interpreting trends in the progression of SDAT.

9-6.   Heston, L.L., Mastri, A.R., Anderson, V.E. & White, J. (1981). Dementia of the Alzheimer type. Archives of General   Psychiatry, 38, 1085-1090.

The study is concerned with exploring the possibility of genetic transmission of Alzheimer's disease since there is evidence that the disease occurs more frequently among siblings and other family members of those individuals who are known to have the disease. Using autopsies and personal data from a group of 2,204 individuals deceased between 1952 and 1972 in Minnesota, 304 cases of primary dementia were identified; 231 of these cases were diagnosed as Dementia of the Alzheimer's Type (DAT) and 73 as other dementias. The study sample was comprised of 125 of the 231 persons identified with DAT. Families were questioned and medical records of these patients examined. Within these families, 87 secondary cases of DAT were found with autopsied verification of DAT in 24 cases. Additionally, 30 of the sample group were identified to have Alzheimer's onset before 65 years of age. Findings indicated that when onset of the disease was earlier, the course was shorter. Also, where there was early onset and a parent had DAT, the probability for DAT in siblings was higher. With early onset cases, there was a greater probability in the family of Down's syndrome and lymphoma, and a higher rate of early mortality, particularly infant mortality.

The findings of the study are very tentative and based on probable association. Much of the medical record keeping of the original sample was incomplete, and was also incomplete for the secondary group. An assumption was made in secondary cases where autopsy was not performed that the individual did have DAT. Although the data obtained are not definitive, the findings of the study would indicate that the probability of generational transmission is greater than chance.

9-7. Husain, M.M. & Nemeroff, C.B. (1990). Neuropeptides and Alzheimer's disease. <u>Journal of the American Geriatric Society</u>, <u>38</u>, 918-925.

The literature regarding the changes in neuropeptides which are associated with Alzheimer's disease is reviewed. Although there are conflicting results in several experiments with various neuropeptides, there is general agreement that somatostatin (SRIF), neuropeptide Y (NPY), cordicotropin-releasing factor (CRF), and vasopressin (AVP) are reduced with Alzheimer's disease, at least in some areas of the brain. It was found that reductions in SRIF are of the greatest magnitude, but there are some inconsistencies in findings, and similar reductions in SRIF are also found in cases of depression and schizophrenia. Therefore, decreases in SRIF cannot be used to identify AD since that neuropeptide is associated with other cognitive dysfunctions.

This is a comprehensive review of experimental results of alteration of neuropeptide-containing neurons in autopsy of individuals diagnosed with Alzheimer's disease. The summary table presented indicates that there is more agreement among experiments and experimental groups with each of the neuropeptides presented than is indicated when the individual findings are discussed by the authors. It would appear that using changes in neuropeptide concentration, at least in cerebrospinal fluid, would not assist in identification of AD, and therefore this method has limited usage as a predictor of the disease.

9-8. Kitwood, T. (1990). The dialectics of dementia: With particular reference to Alzheimer's disease. <u>Ageing and Society</u>, <u>10</u>, 177-196.

As persons suffer losses, their self-esteem is threatened; this loss of self-esteem, along with physical losses, causes them to be treated differently which causes more loss of self-esteem and competence; the process escalates. The author describes caretaker and family behaviors which contribute to the loss of self-esteem which then has the potential to contribute to the symptomatology of Alzheimer's disease. The progress of the disease becomes a self-fulfilling prophecy. The author also tentatively hypothesizes that the stress associated with the feelings of loss of self-esteem and incompetency might be a causative agent of actual physical deterioration. However, the author indicates that this would be empirically unprovable.

There is some evidence to support the effect of self-esteem on competency in adults who are treated as Alzheimer's patients since in some cases an autopsy does not reveal the medical symptoms of the disease. Psychological/social factors, in addition to medical symptomatology, would seem to be areas for further study, particularly since Alzheimer's is not accurately confirmable until death, and conditional confirmation as now constructed would be dependent upon malignant social psychology. There is evidence that the medical aspect of

Alzheimer's, neuropathology, only counts for about 30% of the variance in dementia indicating that other factors are involved. Identification of these other factors and understanding and treating them might make the progress of the disease less difficult for both the patient and the caretaker.

9-9. Mungas, D. (1991). In-office mental status testing: A practical guide. Geriatrics, 46, 54-66.

Basic information regarding the cognitive deficiencies associated with dementia of both irreversible and reversible causation are presented. Emphasis is placed on the importance of early diagnosis of reversible dementias to prevent permanent pathological changes in the brain which occur when causative factors are not remedied. There is a clear presentation of the cognitive deficits associated with dementia and informal screening procedures which may be used to assist diagnosis. Additionally, more specific symptomatology for Alzheimer's Disease, including onset patterns and progression, are included. The final portion of the article presents the Mini-Mental State Examination (MMSE), a gross screening tool useful by primary care physicians to both qualify and quantify impairment due to dementia in a preliminary way. The author emphasizes that the MMSE has limitations which affect its utility as a diagnostic tool.

This is an excellent article which addresses the concerns and needs of primary care physicians, but which is very useful to students/practitioners who desire clearly presented information regarding the symptomatology and diagnosis of dementia. The author includes several very informative tables which provide summary information pertinent to the article, including a summary interpretation for the MMSE scores based on level of impairment. Additionally, the limitations of the MMSE are presented as well as the use of the MMSE as a screening tool. The article is written in a non-technical manner and provides information useful in understanding other more technical, complex literature on dementia, including Alzheimer's Disease.

9-10. Nalbantoglu, J., Lacoste-Royal, G. & Gauvreau, D. (1990). Genetic factors in Alzheimer's disease. Journal of the American Geriatric Society, 38, 564-568.

At this time, twin studies which might affirm genetic inheritance of Alzheimer's disease (AD) have not been completed. However, indications, of genetic influence in AD have come from the association of trisomy 21 or Down's syndrome and AD in families with AD. The incidence of Down's syndrome is slightly higher in families with AD, indicating a possible relationship with chromosome number 21 and the genes located on that chromosome. There are some indications that both late and early onset AD have genetic tendencies and that there is a genetic susceptibility to environmental toxins and/or to infectious agents. Thus far there have been several studies suggestive of linkages to markers on chromosome 21, but there is considerable variability in results which may be attributable to the conditions of the experiments.

The article is a review of previously performed research and presents logical argument based on research studies pertaining to genetic factors which are associated with AD. The authors hypothesize regarding direct inheritance of a gene for AD as well as hypothesizing a genetic susceptibility to environmental and/or infectious agents. There is a summary of recent experiments with genetic markers, particularly the earlier work with chromosome 21. Although presenting no new breakthroughs in experimentation, the authors present support for familial factors and the importance of identification of the gene(s) so that therapeutic modulation of genetic expression might be detained or modified.

9-11. Otsuka, A., Mikami, H., Katahira, K., Nakamoto, Y., Minamitani, K., Imaoka, M., Nishide, M., & Ogihara, T. (1990). Absence of nocturnal fall in blood pressure in elderly persons with Alzheimer-Type dementia. Journal of the American Geriatrics Society, 38, 973-978.

Four groups of elderly Japanese subjects were tested to determine if the circadian rhythm pattern of zenith in the morning and nadir at night of the heart rate and blood pressure were altered in patients who were severely cognitively impaired with probable Alzheimer's Disease. Each of the four groups were diagnosed differently: one group was a normotensive (characterized by normal blood pressure) Alzheimer's group (D), the second was normotensive bedridden patients with orthopedic disorder but without dementia (R), the third was normotensive without dementia with normal daily activity (N), and the fourth group was hypertensive (characterized by high blood pressure) patients with normal daily activity (H). The patients were monitored for 24 hours with a portable automated apparatus which at 30 minute intervals measured and recorded systolic blood pressure, diastolic blood pressure, heart rate, and average blood pressure. Activities of daily living and sleep were also monitored for normalcy over this testing period; irregularities required another 24 hour testing. Findings indicated differences: the N, H, and R groups exhibited normal type circadian rhythms with zenith late in the daytime and nadir between midnight and 4 a.m. The D group did not exhibit the same blood pressure pattern: day and evening averages for diastolic, systolic, and average blood pressure remained relatively constant. However, there was a drop in heart rate in the D group comparable to the other three groups.

In examining the methodology there would seem to be several problems. First, the procedure was performed only once over one twenty-four hour period unless there was some unusual problem occurring. Additionally, each of the four groups consisted of a small sample of only 7-9 subjects. Also, there could be other types of sleep disturbances in the Alzheimer's patients that might affect the results. The tabular data and the graphs which are included indicate each of the four groups and the subtle differences between them. However, the author's conclusion of the study indicates that there is a lack of certainty that the alteration of circadian rhythm of blood pressure found in the Alzheimer's group of patients is related to the effects of Alzheimer's disease.

9-12. Ship, J.A., DeCarli, C., Friedland, R.P., and Baum, B.J. (1990). Diminished submandibular salivary flow in dementia of the Alzheimer type. Journal of Gerontology, 45, M61-M66.

Twenty-six community based older persons suspected of Dementia of the Alzheimer Type (DAT) who were neither taking medication nor had any other psychiatric disorders were paired with a similar group of healthy, age-matched controls who were also part of a study at the National Institute of Aging. The researchers were testing for differences, if any, in salivary flow between the two groups. Results indicated significant differences between the DAT group and the control group in both stimulated and unstimulated submandibular secretion; there were no significant differences in parotid flow rates. Studies have shown that glandular change is a function of age. However, there have been no studies done on changes as a result of Alzheimer's, so it is unknown if additional histological changes in those with DAT occur in addition to normal aging changes. Additionally, there seems to be no neurological explanation for the secretion change; other associated neurological changes which would be caused by damage to the 7th cranial nerve affecting salivary output are not seen.

The methodology of the study may be questioned since the testing procedure was performed only one time and is not a duplication study of other research findings. Therefore, the findings need to be replicated before they are accepted. The authors claim that the implications of the study are of great import for the care of patients with DAT since the hypofunction of the submandibular salivary gland is associated with oral complications; additionally, the addition of psychotropic drugs to treat the DAT would cause additional complications through even further decreased salivary gland output. If there is value to determining the association of salivary gland secretion deficiency with DAT and with oral health, then further testing needs to be completed to verify the results of this study.

9-13. Teri, L. & Wagner, A.W. (1991). Assessment of depression in patients with Alzheimer's Disease: Concordance among informants. Psychology and Aging, 6, 280-285.

The primary focus of this study was to determine if there were differences among clinicians, caregivers, and subjects in assessment of depression levels in Alzheimer's Disease (AD) patients. Based on a sample of 75 patients who had been diagnosed as AD using the criteria of the Diagnostic and Statistical Manual of Mental Disorders (3rd edition, revised), DSM-III-R, and further assessed using the Mini-Mental State Examination (MMSE), the Dementia Rating Scale (DRS) and the Global Deterioration Scale (GDS), the subjects were found to be predominantly mildly to moderately impaired. The DSM-III-R criteria for depression was used to initially identify clinically depressed subjects and the Hamilton Rating Scale for Depression (HAM-D), an instrument which rates subject, caregiver, and clinicians assessments of depression, was further used to determine rater's depression assessments. The primary predictors of depression were changes in interests, suicidal feeling, initial insomnia, middle insomnia, loss of weight, and somatic anxiety. Findings indicate higher levels of depression in those with less education. Additionally, there were statistically significant differences between patient assessments and the caregiver and clinician assessments; the caregiver and clinician assessments were comparable in those diagnosed as depressed. There were also statistically significant differences among the subject, the caregiver, and the clinician of those diagnosed as non-depressed. In all cases, subjects with AD viewed themselves exhibiting lower symptomatology of depression than other assessors. Overall, the level of cognitive impairment did not have an effect on the discrepancies in assessments among the subject, the caregiver, and the clinician.

The findings of this study are comparable to other studies which are cited by the authors. The study methodology is presented and findings supplemented by tables. Overall, this study has been well designed and well executed with both multivariate and univariate statistical measures employed to confirm data outcomes. All statistical manipulations were specified and findings presented. This was an excellent article which was presented in a concise, clear, and readable manner.

9-14. Vitiello, M.V., Prinz, P.N., Williams, D.E., Frommlet, M.S. and Ries, R.K. (1990). Sleep disturbances in patients with mild-stage Alzheimer's disease. Journal of Gerontology, 45, M131-138.

One of the problems medical science is trying to address is finding a way to distinguish Alzheimer's disease from other cognitive type disorders, some of which may be treatable in other ways than is Alzheimer's disease. This study examines sleep patterns of 44 carefully selected mild Alzheimer's probable diagnosed patients and 45 control patients of statistically similar demographic characteristics except for significant differences in age; the control group was younger. Subjects were studied for 72 hours: the first night was an orientation/observational night, and nights two and three were recording nights. Data were collected, interpreted, and averaged for the two nights. Results indicated increases in frequency and duration of awakening and decreases of stages 3 and 4 sleep. However, the results were too inconsistent to separate Alzheimer's patients from the control patients. Other observational studies of Alzheimer patients had indicated Alzheimer Disease (AD) patients were more wakeful and less consistent in sleep patterns. Several studies were reviewed and compared with the less indicative findings of this study of less impaired, mildly affected AD patients. Accurate diagnosis of AD was indicated to be only 63% in mildly affected patients, and this low level of accuracy is not useful for diagnostic purposes. This same method, however, is more accurate (90%) in more severely affected AD patients.

The study methodology was the same as that performed on three other levels of certainly diagnosed AD patients. Repetition of the measures remained adequate, and since this was a replication of previously performed experiments, it indicates that at possible and probably diagnosed AD, the usefulness of sleep patterns for diagnosis of AD is decreased. The age differences between the control and experiment group were covaried out as part of the MANCOVA, so possible age differences in sleep patterns were accounted for. It would seem that since diagnosis is only possible/probable based on National Institute of Neurologic and Communicative Diseases and Stroke/Alzheimer's and Related Disorders Association (NINCDS-ADRDA) criteria, there is less accuracy in the diagnostic categories. It would appear that below the level of mild-moderate AD, this procedure is not useful.

9-15. Wade, J.P.H., Mirsen, T.R., Hachinski, V.C., Fisman, M., Lau, C. & Merskey, H. (1987). The clinical diagnosis of Alzheimer's disease. Archives of Neurology, 44, 24-29.

Sixty-five patients, part of a dementia study of 331 patients, were clinically evaluated prior to death. The assessment included a neurological evaluation which provided an ischemic score (IS) used to differentiate different types of dementia, a psychological assessment, a serial electroencephalogram, and a CT scan (in all but five cases). A clinical diagnosis was undertaken by a neurologist using the data available, except for autopsy data, on each of the subjects. The clinical assessment placed each patient into one of four categories: degenerative dementia of the Alzheimer's type (DAT), multi-infarct dementia (MID), mixed DAT and multi-infarct dementia, and other specific diagnosis. Conclusions were based on specific criteria from each of the measures taken. The results of these clinical diagnoses were compared with autopsy findings based on morphometric diagnosis. The results indicated that although the measures used clinically were not totally accurate, they could be utilized with relative confidence of accuracy with those elderly patients with moderate to severe Alzheimer disease. The most error in diagnosis was in the mixed group where only 5 of 16 patients were determined to be mixed upon autopsy. According to the authors, the ischemic scale score did not discriminate well between multi-infarct dementia and those with both multi-infarct dementia and DAT, the mixed group.

The study explores the reliability of the IS as a diagnostic tool through comparison of diagnosis based on autopsy. The study is well designed, but indicates that the implementation of the IS is dependent upon the skill of the diagnostician in the clinical setting. The IS, particularly with some revision and refinement, may become a useful tool for diagnosis of Alzheimer's disease in community patients.

10

APOLIPOPROTEINS AND CORONARY HEART DISEASE

John Contois

INTRODUCTION

Coronary heart disease (CHD) is responsible for more than 500,000 deaths in the U.S. each year; more deaths annually than any other disease including all forms of cancer combined. There are several risk factors that may lead to heart disease, including: elevated serum cholesterol level, hypertension, cigarette smoking, diabetes mellitus, obesity, and family history of CHD. It is less appreciated that age is a risk factor as well. CHD is the major cause of death in the elderly, and three out of four CHD deaths occur in people over age 65. Morbidity due to heart disease is also considerable in this age group. Data from the Framingham Heart Study and other clinical studies show a high prevalence of heart disease in the elderly, many of whom are asymptomatic and otherwise fit. Despite the fact that chronic diseases, such as CHD, are essentially diseases afflicting the aged, few studies have focused on this population.

Cholesterol and other lipids serve important roles in normal physiology. Cholesterol is an essential component of cell membranes and serves as a precursor of bile acids (required for fat absorption), adrenal steroids, and sex hormones. Other lipids, such as triglycerides and phospholipids, are also important in cell membranes and as precursors to certain hormones and prostaglandins. Metabolically, dietary lipids are a concentrated source of energy and may have a sparing effect on protein. The transport of lipids in the blood requires that they be packaged into a particle in such a way that the hydrophilic ("water-loving") constituents are arranged on the outside of the particle and the hydrophobic ("water-fearing") components stay in the core. In addition to lipids these particles also contain one or more characteristic proteins, called apolipoproteins (apos), and are therefore referred to as lipoprotein particles. The core of these particles contain triglyceride and cholesterol (cholesteryl esters) while the outer shell is comprised of phospholipids, unesterified cholesterol, and apolipoproteins.

Lipoproteins are commonly classified by their physical and chemical properties, such as density, electrophoretic mobility, size and composition. The most familiar classification is based on density: chylomicrons, very low density lipoprotein (VLDL), low density lipoprotein (LDL), and high density lipoprotein (HDL). These particles have very different compositions and are physiologically distinct. The largest and least dense particles are chylomicrons. These triglyceride-rich particles are synthesized by the intestine following a high fat meal. VLDL are also rich in triglyceride and are secreted by the liver following the uptake of chylomicron remnants. LDL particles, secreted by the liver or formed from VLDL, are the major carriers of cholesterol in the bloodstream and contain apo B. Elevated levels of LDL cholesterol are considered atherogenic. HDL, which contain apo AI as their major apolipoprotein, are cholesterol-rich particles involved in reverse cholesterol transport, the removal of cholesterol from peripheral tissues back to the liver for excretion or reuse, and are thought to be protective against CHD. Lipoprotein (a) [Lp(a)] is an LDL-like particle with an extra apolipoprotein, apo(a), covalently bound to the apo B of LDL. An elevated level of Lp(a) has been shown to be a strong, independent risk factor for coronary heart disease in a number of case-control studies. Unlike other lipoproteins, Lp(a) concentration is not influenced by diet, but it appears to correlate strongly with family history of premature heart disease. Lipoproteins play a central role in cholesterol transport and risk of CHD. The importance of LDL- and HDL-cholesterol, in addition to serum total cholesterol, as cardiovascular risk factors is clearly established. This same relationship between total and lipoprotein cholesterol levels and CHD risk has also been observed in elderly subjects.

Regulation of these lipoprotein particles is largely mediated by surface apolipoproteins which activate a number of enzymes involved in lipid metabolism and serve as ligands for binding to tissues. Apolipoproteins have been referred to, therefore, as the "business end" of the lipoprotein particle. It is reasonable, then, to suppose that levels of serum apolipoproteins, as well as serum cholesterol, are predictive of CHD, and this has in fact been demonstrated. Apos also provide a measure of the total number of atherogenic particles in the circulation; since there is only one molecule of apo B per lipoprotein particle, apo B concentration provides a measure of the total number of VLDL and LDL particles in the circulation. Intuitively, it is reasonable to expect measurement of apolipoproteins to provide an assessment of CHD risk independent of lipoprotein cholesterol measurement, despite the obvious correlation of these two parameters. The interrelationship of apolipoproteins with other lipid risk factors poses a number of methodological and statistical problems, and determining the degree to which these parameters are related is tied to the question of whether apolipoprotein measurement improves our ability to predict CHD risk. Some researchers would argue that the relationship of apos with CHD is secondary to the association of apos with lipoprotein cholesterol level. Nevertheless, apolipoproteins are direct gene products and, at least in terms of the genetic component of risk, should provide insights beyond what is provided by cholesterol measurement alone.

Genetic variability of apolipoproteins, as assessed by isoelectric focusing (IEF) and restriction fragment length polymorphism (RFLP) techniques, is also shown to influence serum lipid concentrations, and certain phenotypes are seen more frequently in individuals with CHD compared with control subjects. IEF followed by immunoblotting has become the standard technique for determining apo E phenotype. In humans, apo E has three common isoforms, apo E2, E3, and E4, which differ by an amino acid substitution at two sites along the 299-amino acid chain. Apo E3, the most common form of the protein, contains cysteine at site 112 and arginine at site 158, while apo E2 has cysteine at both sites and apo E4 has arginine at both sites. This small difference in the protein gives apo E4 an additional positive charge relative to apo E3, which in turn has an additional positive charge compared to apo E2. This feature gives the three isoforms different isoelectric points, which allows phenotype to be determined by isoelectric focusing, a technique whereby a protein travels along a pH gradient under the influence of an electric current until it reaches its isoelectric point. Use of this procedure has shown apo E polymorphism to have a strong influence on plasma cholesterol levels. RFLP, which detects changes in the nucleotide sequence of DNA, has not provided any consistent data relative to apolipoproteins and CHD risk. Theoretically, if these DNA alterations occur in regions coding for an apolipoprotein, then the metabolism of that protein may be altered. The procedure is relatively straightforward; purified DNA is digested with an enzyme (restriction endonuclease) that recognizes a certain nucleotide sequence and cleaves the DNA at a specific point. The resulting DNA fragments are separated by size using electrophoresis. Polymorphisms are identified from the characteristic fragments. Other apolipoproteins such as apo AII, AIV, CII, and CIII are less well understood although they all appear to play important roles in the metabolism of lipoproteins.

This bibliography represents a comprehensive review of recent articles dealing with the association of apolipoproteins and coronary heart disease in human subjects. I excluded review articles, letters, and editorials except where new data were presented or, in my opinion, the information was particularly important. The majority of studies are case-control studies with myocardial infarction (MI) patients or subjects with angiographic evidence of significant atherosclerotic disease. For the most part, apo AI and apo B concentrations and/or polymorphisms were the focus of these articles. It is evident from these data that apolipoproteins are involved in the development of CHD, and measurement of apolipoproteins appears to be useful in assessing risk of cardiovascular disease. The notable exception is the article by Stampfer et al., the sole prospective study among the recent literature, who report no additional benefit from the measurement of apos AI and B. In the case-control studies, however, which argue less forcefully than prospective data, apolipoproteins AI and B appear to be better markers for CHD than HDL- and LDL-cholesterol levels. Also, lipoprotein (a) level is confirmed to be a strong, independent risk factor for CHD in case-control studies. A few articles, focusing on the mechanism of atherosclerosis, studying coronary vessel biopsy samples, show apolipoprotein B and apo(a) to be intimately involved in the process of cholesterol deposition in arterial wall. On the other hand, polymorphism of apolipoproteins as assessed by RFLP prove to be of little value in assessing heart disease risk.

There are a number of factors that can affect the results of lipid and apolipoprotein measurement and make the interpretation of data difficult. Biological, behavioral, and sample handling variables all come into play in influencing lipid measurement; sometimes with dramatic results. It is important to keep in mind that there is no definitive or standardized methods for apolipoprotein measurement, and assay variability between labs and even within labs can be great. Imprecision and inaccuracy in apolipoprotein measurements, if present in a study, would be expected to weaken the associations between these values and CHD. Therefore, when an adequately controlled study shows positive results the data are probably valid. A lack of association between apolipoprotein variables and CHD, on the other hand, may reflect the quality of the assays. It is also important to keep in mind that with retrospective studies CHD patients may have been advised to make lifestyle changes that may weaken the association of lipids and CHD. Medication use is carefully controlled in most studies, but drugs and diet are potential confounding variables.

In summary, it is clear from these data that apolipoproteins and Lp(a) are directly involved in the process of atherosclerosis. Whether or not apo AI and/or apo B measurement improves our ability to assess CHD risk is less clear, however.

ANNOTATED BIBLIOGRAPHY

10-1. Acoltzin, C., and Lezama, Y. (1990). Lack of apolipoprotein AI in patients recovering from myocardial infarction. The American Journal of Cardiology, 66, 124.

In a brief report the authors describe their study of 16 subjects with previous myocardial infarction (MI) and 44 control subjects apparently free of disease. Blood apolipoprotein AI levels were determined by an immunodiffusion technique. The patient group had significantly lower apo AI levels than controls. These data show apo AI to be a potentially useful marker for assessing CHD risk.

10-2. Al-Muhtaseb, N., Hayat, N., and Al-Khafaji, M. (1989). Lipoproteins and apolipoproteins in young male survivors of myocardial infarction. Atherosclerosis, 77, 131-138.

This study investigated plasma lipids, lipoproteins, and apolipoproteins in young, male survivors of myocardial infarction. Subjects were 60 males, aged 28-40 years, admitted to a cardiac care unit following MI. Diagnosis was based on chest pain of at least 30 minutes duration, electrocardiographic evidence of infarction, and enzyme profiles characteristic of MI. Control subjects were matched for age, height, body weight, and family history of MI. Fasting blood was drawn at 10 days and 4 months after MI for plasma analysis of total cholesterol, triglycerides, phospholipids, and apolipoproteins AI, AII, and B. Density fractions were collected after sequential ultracentrifugation for VLDL, LDL, HDL, HDL_2 and HDL_3 for lipid analyses. The apolipoproteins were measured by radial immunodiffusion; cholesterol, triglycerides, and phospholipids were measured enzymatically.

There were no differences between control and patient groups with respect to mean age, body mass index (BMI), blood pressure, level of exercise, smoking, or family history of MI. There were also no differences between patients' lipid parameters at 10 days and at 4 months. MI patients had higher levels of total cholesterol, LDL-cholesterol, total triglycerides, VLDL-triglycerides, LDL-triglycerides, HDL-triglycerides, phospholipids, apo B, and LDL-apo B; and lower levels of HDL-cholesterol, HDL_2-cholesterol, apo AI, and HDL-apo AI. In MI survivors apo AI correlated positively with HDL-cholesterol and negatively with total and LDL-triglycerides. Stepwise discriminant analysis between controls and MI survivors at 4 months shows that the best discriminators between the two groups are plasma levels of HDL_2-cholesterol, apo B, apo AI, VLDL-triglycerides, HDL-cholesterol, and plasma triglycerides, in this order. Using these parameters 92% of the patients and 90% of the controls were correctly classified. Therefore, apolipoproteins AI and B, and HDL_2-cholesterol appear to be useful markers of CAD risk.

10-3. Barbir, M., Wile, D., Trayer, I., Aber, V.R., and Thompson, G.R. (1988). High prevalence of hypertriglyceridaemia and apolipoprotein abnormalities in coronary artery disease. British Heart Journal, 60, 397-403.

Serum lipids and apolipoproteins AI and B were measured in 174 men less than age 60 with coronary artery disease as confirmed by angiography. Subjects were non-diabetic, not taking lipid lowering medications, and without previous history of myocardial infarct or bypass surgery, and they had greater than 50% stenosis of at least one coronary artery. Control subjects were 572 healthy men between the ages of 20-60 with normal electrocardiograms. Lipids were measured enzymatically, apo AI was determined immunoturbidimetrically, and apo B was measured by radialimmunodiffusion.

CAD patients had higher mean values for serum total cholesterol, triglycerides, LDL-cholesterol, and LDL-apolipoprotein B; and lower mean values for HDL-cholesterol and apolipoprotein AI compared to control subjects. CAD patients also had a higher frequency of high LDL-apo B levels and low apo AI levels than controls, with less overlap between patients and controls than with respective LDL and HDL-cholesterol concentrations. Stepwise discriminant function analysis indicated that serum triglyceride was the best discriminator between patients and controls, followed by HDL-cholesterol. Adding apolipoproteins to the model puts apo B in second place, followed by apo AI, which eliminated HDL-cholesterol from the model altogether. This study confirms that apolipoproteins are important markers for CAD, and emphasizes the importance of hypertriglyceridemia as a risk factor, which, at least in this study, was the most important determinant.

10-4. Bondjers, G., Linden, T., Fager, G., Olofsson, S.-O., Olsson, G., and Wiklund, O. (1988). Aortic intimal lipid content and serum lipoproteins in patients undergoing coronary by-pass surgery as related to clinical prognosis. Atherosclerosis, 72, 231-23.

Aortic intimal lipids and apolipoproteins were measured in patients undergoing coronary bypass surgery to assess their predictive value in prognosis. Aortic biopsies were obtained from 37 males undergoing bypass surgery due to severe angina; four were hyperlipidemic, one was diabetic, 68% had a history of sustained myocardial infarction, and 31% were hypertensive. Blood samples were obtained preoperatively for measurement of serum cholesterol, triglycerides, HDL-cholesterol, and apolipoproteins AI, AII, and B.

Free and esterified cholesterol, triglycerides, lecithin, and sphingomyelin were found in the intimal biopsies, and there was a strong correlation between free and esterified cholesterol in the tissue. There were positive correlations between serum apo AII and the tissue level of lecithin. Patients with hypertension had significantly higher levels of cholesteryl ester in the intima. Also, there was a correlation between the number of stenosed arteries and serum triglycerides, and an inverse correlation between the number of stenosed arteries and HDL-cholesterol, although there were no correlations of apo AI or AII and atherosclerosis. Apo AI levels did, however, predict prognosis 5 years after surgery; patients with lower AI levels had more severe angina and two subjects had died.

10-5. Bovet, P., Dariol, R., Essinger, A., Golay, A., Sigwart, U., and Kappenberger, L. (1989). Phospholipids and other lipids in angiographically assessed coronary artery disease. Atherosclerosis, 80, 41-47.

This study examined the relationship between angiographically assessed CAD and blood lipids and lipoproteins with particular attention to phospholipid species. Subjects were 114 men, aged 31-73, undergoing angiography for suspected CAD who were classified based on the degree of stenosis; 28 patients without important CAD were compared to 76 patients with significant CAD. Blood was obtained from each subject for serum lipid determinations including phospholipids, triglycerides, total cholesterol, free cholesterol, and apolipoproteins AI and B.

The subjects with CAD had significantly higher levels of total cholesterol, free cholesterol, LDL-cholesterol, phospholipids, LDL-triglycerides and apo B; and lower levels of HDL-cholesterol and HDL_2-cholesterol compared to subjects without CAD. CAD patients also had higher triglycerides and lower apo AI concentrations, but these differences did not quite reach significance. One-variable discriminant functions, measured in order to test the ability of each of the lipid parameters to classify patients with or without CAD, showed that only the apo AI/apo B ratio could achieve a prediction of CAD in greater than 70% of the patients. Free cholesterol/HDL-cholesterol, LDL-cholesterol/ HDL-cholesterol, total cholesterol, phospholipids/HDL-phospholipids, and total cholesterol/HDL-cholesterol could all predict the absence of disease with greater than 70% accuracy. In summary, the apo AI/apo B ratio could accurately classify patients with CAD, but serum phospholipids did not prove to be better predictors of CAD than other lipids.

10-6. Chivot, L., Mainard, F., Bigot, E., Bard, J.M., Auget, J.L., Madec, Y., and Fruchart, J.C. (1990). Logistic discriminant analysis of lipids and apolipoproteins in a population of coronary bypass patients and the significance of apolipoproteins C-III and E. Atherosclerosis, 82, 205-211.

Hypertriglyceridemia as a risk factor for heart disease is still being debated. This article describes a study of apolipoproteins involved in the metabolism of triglyceride-rich particles in patients undergoing coronary bypass surgery and a control group (74 patients and 78 controls, all men). Cholesterol and triglycerides were measured by standard enzymatic methods, and apolipoproteins AI and B were analyzed by immunonephelometry. Apolipoproteins C-III and E were assayed by enzyme-linked immunosorbent assay (ELISA). Apo B-containing particles were separated from other lipoproteins by concanavalin A treatment.

Bypass patients had higher plasma concentrations of total cholesterol, triglycerides, apo B, LDL-cholesterol, and lower HDL-cholesterol and apo AI than controls. Apo E concentration was also higher in patients than controls in both apo B-containing and non-apo B particles. Apo C-III was also significantly higher in patients, but only in the apo B containing particles. Interestingly, there was a significant correlation between triglycerides and both apo C-III and apo E, especially in lipoprotein B particles. Stepwise regression analysis showed that apo C-III measured in apo B-containing particles is more powerful than triglyceride and apo B in discriminating the coronary bypass group, and the addition of apo C-III and apo E serve to better classify individuals in both groups. Therefore, the addition of apolipoproteins of triglyceride-rich lipoproteins provides more information in assessing the risk of coronary heart disease.

10-7. Coste-Burel, M., Mainard, F., Chivot, L., Auget, J.L., and Madec, Y. (1990). Study of lipoprotein particles LpAI and LPAI:AII in patients before coronary bypass surgery. Clinical Chemistry, 36, 1889-1891.

Apo AI and apo AII are two essential proteins in HDL particles. It is believed by many that the HDL particles that protect against CAD are the particles that contain apo AI only (LpAI) and not particles that contain both apo AI and apo AII (LpAI:AII). These two particles could have different metabolic functions. Therefore, the investigators compared lipids, apolipoproteins, and Lp AI and Lp AI:AII levels between CAD patients and healthy control subjects. Forty-three men, mean age 51, hospitalized for coronary bypass surgery were compared to 54 healthy men, mean age 46, recruited from the hospital and university staff. Health was confirmed from history, normal electrocardiogram, absence of angina, and absence of diabetes and other disorders. Patients taking lipid lowering medications were excluded from the study.

Lp AI and Lp AI:AII concentrations were both significantly lower in CAD patients compared to controls. Apo AI correlated with Lp AI and Lp AI:AII in controls but not in patients; Lp AI:AII, and not Lp AI, correlated with apo AI in bypass patients. Discriminant analysis showed that apo AI was the most powerful discriminator between patients and controls, and the addition of Lp AI and Lp AI:AII did not improve the model. Therefore, the authors conclude that the determination of Lp AI and Lp AI:AII particles does not add to lipid and apoprotein measures in assessing CAD risk.

10-8. Cushing, G.L., Gaubatz, J.W., Nava, M.L., Burdick, B.J., Bocan, T.M.A., Guyton, J.R., Weilbaecher, D., DeBakey, M.E., Lawrie, G.M., and

Morrisett, J.D. (1989). Quantitation and localization of apolipoproteins [a] and B in coronary artery bypass vein grafts resected at re-operation. Arteriosclerosis, 9, 593-603.

In this study the role of apolipoproteins (a) and B in atherogenesis is investigated by looking for correlations between plasma and tissue levels of these proteins and the immunochemical localization of apos B and (a) in saphenous vein bypass grafts resected at the time of a second bypass operation. Patients undergoing coronary re-bypass surgery were selected for the study, and segments of saphenous vein grafts and normal saphenous veins (controls) were obtained. Blood was drawn for lipid analyses immediately before or up to 12 hours before surgery. Histological evaluations were made on this fresh tissue, and flash frozen segments were used for immunochemical localization of apolipoproteins. Plasma lipid concentrations were compared to previously reported normal values.

There was no difference in plasma total cholesterol concentration between the patient group and the normal population, but the patient group had a significantly lower mean HDL-cholesterol level and significantly higher plasma triglycerides, Lp(a), and apo B levels. Lesions from six patients were examined for apo(a) and apo B localization. Staining patterns showed that these two proteins co-localized and that they were associated with lipid deposition as determined by general lipid staining. Staining of control grafts showed little or no reaction. Positive correlations were seen between plasma levels of apos B and (a) and their respective tissue levels, and between tissue apo(a) and tissue apo B. Tissue apo B was also correlated with morphological measurements of atherosclerosis, providing further support for apo(a) and apo B involvement in arterial disease progression.

10-9. Dorow, D.S., Burke, J., and Goding, J.W. (1989). Assessment of a PstI polymorphism of the apolipoprotein-AI gene in Australian patients with coronary artery disease. Australian and New Zealand Journal of Medicine, 19, 677-681.

This study addressed the usefulness of a PstI restriction fragment length polymorphism of the apo AI gene as a marker for heart disease risk in an Australian population. In previous studies a 3.3 kb fragment from PstI digested DNA was found to be strongly associated with premature CAD. Blood was collected from 200 coronary patients of whom 100 had definitive CAD. Ninety-three control samples were obtained from hospital staff members and from a Red Cross blood bank. DNA was extracted, digested with PstI, electrophoresed in agarose, and blotted. After probing with a radiolabelled apo AI probe, bands were visualized by autoradiography.

Interestingly, the control group proved to have the highest frequency of the 3.3 kb allele- not the patient group as expected. This illustrates the ambiguous results often seen with RFLP methodology.

10-10. Durrington, P.N., Ishola, M., Hunt, L., Arrol, S., and Bhatnagar, D. (1988). Apolipoproteins (a), AI, and B and parental history in men with early onset ischemic heart disease. Lancet, 881 (8594), 1070-1073.

Apolipoproteins AI, B, and a parental history of heart disease as risk factors for heart disease were assessed in 48 patients and 82 control subjects, all men, in Manchester, England. Patients with definite evidence of myocardial infarction admitted to the cardiac care unit served as subjects; controls were healthy men from similar social backgrounds with no history of ischemic heart disease. Serum apo B and apo AI were measured with an immunoradiometric assay.

The authors found a significant difference between patients and controls for serum apo B, apo AI, VLDL-cholesterol, and HDL-cholesterol concentrations. Serum apo(a) was higher in patients, but the difference was not quite significant. Interestingly, while apo B levels were higher in patients, there was no difference in LDL-cholesterol. Discriminant analysis showed that apo AI and apo B and a knowledge of parental history of early cardiac death were the best predictors of myocardial infarction. Apo(a) could substitute for parental history in the model, supporting the theory that apo(a) is a reliable genetic marker for CAD.

The authors do not describe their methodology or assay variability. However, they carefully controlled for age, BMI, blood pressure, alcohol consumption, and physical exercise; factors that may affect lipids but are usually overlooked.

10-11. Eche, Y., Azema, C., De Graeve, J., Valdiguie, P.M., Bouissou, H. and Fievet, C. (1990). Microdetermination of cutaneous apoprotein B: Application to screening of coronary heart disease. Clinical Chemistry, 36, 576-577.

The authors have developed a method for determining apolipoprotein B concentration from skin biopsies which they suggest can be an additional tool for the early detection of coronary heart disease. The advantages are that the skin punch biopsy requires a very small sample and is relatively easy to perform. Their data suggests that skin apo B may be a more sensitive indicator than serum apo B for CHD, but comparisons to other lipid risk factors are not made. More research is necessary to confirm and validate this new methodology.

10-12. Eto, M., Watanabe, K., and Makino, I. (1989). Increased frequencies of apolipoprotein E2 and E4 alleles in patients with ischemic heart disease.

Clinical Genetics, <u>36</u>, 183-188.

It has been established that apo E polymorphism is associated with atherosclerosis, although the exact relationship of different alleles is still controversial. Eto et al., therefore, examined apo E alleles and coronary heart disease in Japanese subjects. Patients with CHD, 55 males and 54 females, were compared to 576 control subjects, 422 male, from the same geographic area as the patients. Plasma total cholesterol, triglycerides, HDL-cholesterol, VLDL-cholesterol, and VLDL-triglycerides were determined. Apo E phenotypes were determined from the VLDL density fraction by isoelectric focusing and immunoblotting.

Both apo E2-present phenotypes (apos E 3/2, E 2/2, E 4/2) and apo E4-present phenotypes (apos E 4/3, E 4/4, E 4/2) were significantly more frequent in the CHD patients than in the control population. This study supports previous reports that the E4 allele is associated with higher cholesterol levels and atherosclerosis. Apo E2, on the other hand, has previously been found to be neutral or even antiatherogenic. Perhaps there are cross-cultural differences, both genetic and environmental, that relate to the difference seen with this Japanese population.

10-13. Ford, E.S., Cooper, R.S., Simmons, B., and Castaner, A. (1990). Serum lipids, lipoproteins, and apolipoproteins in Black patients with angiographically defined coronary artery disease. <u>Journal of Clinical Epidemiology</u>, <u>43</u>, 425-432.

This article is especially noteworthy because the subjects of this research were blacks with angiographically defined coronary artery disease. All previous studies with a similar objective have used predominantly white male subjects. Subjects were 151 men and 245 women with 70% or greater narrowing of at least one coronary artery or greater than 50% stenosis of the left main coronary artery. These individuals were compared to others with atherosclerotic vessels less than 50% stenosed. Total cholesterol, LDL-cholesterol, HDL-cholesterol, LDL-cholesterol/HDL-cholesterol ratio, triglycerides, apolipoproteins AI and B, and the apo AI/B ratio were determined. Apolipoproteins were measured by immunodiffusion.

Significant differences were found between cases and controls for total cholesterol, HDL-cholesterol, triglycerides, LDL-cholesterol, apo AI and apo B for women; in men no significant differences were found, although the trends were the same. Using a stepwise regression analysis only the ratio of apo AI/B was associated with disease in women; no parameters were associated with CAD in men. Overall, the apo AI/B ratio appears to be the best predictor of CAD in this population.

The lack of any associations between lipids and CAD is surprising. A major flaw of this study may be the comparison of cases and controls based on the degree of stenosis of the major arteries. Individuals with less than 50% stenosis may still be in the early stages of disease. Also, age and other risk factors are not controlled.

10-14. Genest, J.J., Ordovas, J.M., McNamara, J.R., Robbins, T.M., Cohn, S.D., Salem, D.N., Wilson, P.W.F., Masharani, U., Frossard, P.M., and Schaefer, E.J. (1990). DNA polymorphisms of the apolipoprotein B gene in patients with premature coronary artery disease. Atherosclerosis, 82, 7-17.

The authors looked at restriction fragment length polymorphisms of the apo B gene to see if genetic variability within this gene may contribute to heart disease risk. The subjects were 111 white males with premature coronary artery disease as assessed by angiography and 122 elderly white males free of cardiovascular disease as assessed by a lack of clinical signs and symptoms and electrocardiogram abnormalities. Allele frequency of four RFLPs within the apo B gene were compared in these two populations. The authors chose an elderly control group to maximize the likelihood of finding a difference in the frequencies of the different polymorphisms. Lipids and lipoprotein cholesterol levels were determined by standardized enzymatic assays, and apos B and AI were measured by ELISA. RFLPs were determined using four restriction endonucleases: MspI (at two sites), EcoRI, XbaI, and PvuII.

There were significant differences between patients and controls with regard to plasma total cholesterol, triglycerides, LDL-cholesterol, HDL-cholesterol, and apo AI; the controls had higher levels for all of the above except for triglycerides, which were lower. There were interesting and significant differences seen with the MspI insertion polymorphism and with the EcoRI polymorphism between the CAD and control groups, but not with XbaI and PvuII. The authors point out that even though there is a significant difference between CAD patients and control subjects, the value of RFLPs as a screening tool is limited since traditional lipid values provide relatively more information about CAD risk.

10-15. Grundy, S.M., and Vega, G.L. (1990). Role of apolipoprotein levels in clinical practice (Editorial). Archives of Internal Medicine, 150, 1579-1582.

This editorial discusses the potential for apolipoprotein measurement as a tool for assessing CAD risk. It also provides a fairly complete and accurate review of the different methodologies currently being used to measure apolipoproteins and their flaws. The article points out that there are not, as yet, validated and standardized techniques for the determination of apolipoproteins

AI or B. The current optimism for the use of apolipoprotein measurement in a clinical setting to assess heart disease risk must be tempered by the realization that the usefulness of these assays is limited by potential inaccuracies and imprecision.

10-16. Hajjar, K.A., Gavish, D., Breslow, J.L., and Nachman, R.L. (1989). Lipoprotein(a) modulation of endothelial cell surface fibrinolysis and its potential role in atherosclerosis. Nature, 339, 303-305.

The focus of this article was the effect of Lp(a) on the fibrinolytic system in cultured endothelial cells. The authors found that Lp(a) interferes with fibrinolysis by inhibiting plasminogen binding. Plasminogen binding is important in the breakdown of clots and the development of lesions. A second aspect of this article is the demonstration of Lp(a) accumulation in atherosclerotic lesions, taken from autopsy samples. Using immunohistochemical techniques with a monospecific polyclonal antibody against human Lp(a), they compared vessels from normal and diseased tissue. They report a striking accumulation of Lp(a) in atherosclerotic coronary arteries and no detectable binding of anti-Lp(a) in normal coronary vessels from another subject.

Since this was a secondary aspect of the research this data and methodology are not discussed in great detail. Apparently, only two subjects were studied: one with CAD and one without. This study shows, that Lp(a) interacts with arterial endothelial cells and supports the notion of a direct link between serum Lp(a) concentration and atherosclerotic heart disease.

10-17. Hong, M.L., James, R.W., Grab, B., and Pometta, D. (1988). High density lipoprotein (HDL) subfractions in cardiovascular patients with low levels of HDL-cholesterol: Influence of hypertriglyceridemia on subfraction concentration and composition. Atherosclerosis, 69, 241-248.

It is well documented that HDL-cholesterol levels are important determinants of coronary artery disease risk. This study examines the lipid composition of HDL subfractions in CAD patients to define this association more clearly. Male patients with angiographic evidence of atherosclerosis were screened for plasma HDL-cholesterol and triglyceride levels. Subjects were assigned to 3 groups: individuals with HDL-cholesterol levels below the 20th percentile and triglycerides above the 95th percentile, based on the Geneva, Switzerland population, were assigned to Group 1; normotriglyceridemic CAD patients with HDL-cholesterol below the 20th percentile were assigned to Group 2; while group 3 was a control group comprised of age-matched, healthy individuals with HDL-cholesterol levels above the 20th percentile and plasma triglycerides below the 90th percentile. Fasting blood was separated into lipoprotein subclasses by ultracentrifugation. Lipids were measured enzymatically and apolipoproteins were determined by electroimmunoassay.

There were no differences between patients and controls with respect to plasma total cholesterol, and there were no differences between group 2 (normal triglycerides) and controls with respect to BMI, but the high triglyceride group had a significantly higher mean BMI. As selected, both patients groups had lower HDL-cholesterol levels compared to controls. The major HDL_2 components, total protein and phospholipids, were significantly lower in both groups of patients compared to controls, while there were no differences between the two patient groups. Within the HDL_3 subfraction, the patient groups again had significantly lower levels of total protein and phospholipids. The high triglyceride patient group also had significantly higher levels of triglyceride in this subfraction compared to controls and the other patient group. Apo AI was significantly lower than controls in HDL_2 and HDL_3 subfractions in the high-triglyceride patient group, but not in the normotriglyceridemic group.

This article illustrates the relationship between BMI and plasma triglycerides, and also shows the importance of plasma triglycerides in influencing HDL subfraction composition and CAD risk.

10-18. Kuusi, T., Nieminen, M.S., Ehnholm, C., Yki-Jarvinen, H., Valle, M., Nikkila, E.A., and Taskinen, M.-R. (1989). Apoprotein E polymorphism and coronary artery disease: Increased prevalence of apolipoprotein E-4 in angiographically verified coronary patients. Arteriosclerosis, 9, 237-241.

Apo E phenotype frequencies were compared between 91 men with angiographically confirmed coronary artery disease and the Finnish population in general (previously published survey data). Cholesterol and triglycerides were measured in serum using standard enzymatic methods; apo AI and apo AII were determined by immunoturbidimetry, and apo B was determined by immunodiffusion. Apo E phenotypes were determined by isoelectric focusing.

The authors report a distribution of apo E-phenotypes among the CAD patients that is different from the expected frequencies. There was a significant increase in E 4/4 and E 4/3 phenotypes and a significant decrease in E 3/3 in CAD patients. This was independent of age and the severity of heart disease. As expected, there was an increase in LDL-cholesterol and apo B concentrations in individuals with the E-4 phenotypes, both patients and controls. There were no other differences in lipid parameters between apo E-phenotypes. This report confirms other studies showing a link between the apo E-4 allele and CAD risk.

10-19. Linden, T., Bondjers, G., Fager, G., Olofsson, S.-O., and Wiklund, O. (1989). Apolipoprotein B in human aortic biopsies in relation to serum lipids and lipoproteins. Atherosclerosis, 77, 159-166.

This report describes the relationship between intimal apolipoprotein B from human aortic biopsies and serum lipids. Biopsy samples were obtained from the aorta during coronary bypass surgery from 46 patients, aged 39-71 years. Sixty-three percent of these patients had previously suffered a myocardial infarction and 48% were hyperlipidemic. Fasting blood was obtained before the surgery for measurement of serum cholesterol, triglycerides, and HDL-cholesterol; and apoproteins AI and B, measured by electroimmunoassay. Apo B in the intima was measured by immunoradiometric assay after dissection from the media, washing, and incubation in Tris buffer. Apo B was determined in this "buffer-extractable" fraction and after collagenase digestion of the residual tissue.

Forty-seven percent of the patients had high serum apo B levels and 51% had low HDL-cholesterol levels, defined as greater than the 90th percentile for apo B or less than the 10th percentile for HDL-cholesterol from previously reported normal ranges. The biopsies showed intimal thickening but no plaques. Total intimal apo B was 228 ± 227 $\mu g/g$ wet weight, and there were significant correlations between intimal apo B and serum cholesterol, triglycerides, apo B and LDL-cholesterol. Serum HDL-cholesterol and apo AI did not correlate with tissue apo B. Also, there were no significant correlations between intimal apo B and smoking, hypertension, or previous myocardial infarction. Patients were followed up about 35 months after the initial surgery and classified based on symptoms of angina and surgery outcome. Patients with the best prognosis had significantly higher levels of apo AI and HDL-cholesterol.

The finding of a correlation between apo B, total cholesterol, and LDL-cholesterol in serum and intima apo B strongly suggest that LDL particles, mediated by apo B, are directly involved in lipid deposition in the arterial wall.

10-20. Mendis, S., Shepherd, J., Packard, C.J., and Gaffney, D. (1990). Genetic variation in the cholesteryl ester transfer protein and apolipoprotein A-I genes and its relation to coronary heart disease in a Sri Lankan population. Atherosclerosis, 83, 137-146.

Variation in the cholesteryl ester transfer protein (CETP) gene and in the apolipoprotein AI gene in relation to CAD risk was investigated. CETP is responsible for the exchange of cholesteryl esters between lipoprotein particles in the circulation, and is thought to play a role in cholesterol homeostasis. Ninety-five Sri Lankan male patients with coronary heart disease, confirmed by medical history and electrocardiograms, were compared to an equal number of healthy control subjects. Patients on beta-blockers and anti-hypertensive medications were excluded from the study. Blood was drawn for plasma analysis of total cholesterol, HDL-cholesterol, and triglycerides, all measured by enzymatic methods. 5 μg samples of isolated DNA were digested with TaqI and SstI restriction enzymes and electrophoresed on agarose gels for Southern blotting.

There were no significant differences in the frequency of alleles for TaqIA, TaqIB, or SstI polymorphisms between patients and controls. Also, total cholesterol and triglyceride levels did not show any relation to any of these polymorphisms, although there was a trend for lower HDL-cholesterol levels in control subjects with the B1 allele of the TaqI RFLP. Therefore, these RFLPs do not appear to be useful in assessing CHD risk.

10-21. Niendorf, A., Rath, M., Wolf, K., Peters, S., Arps, H., Beisiegel, U., and Dietel, M. (1990). Morphological detection and quantification of lipoprotein(a) deposition in atheromatous lesions of human aorta and coronary arteries. Virchows Archives of Pathological Anatomy and Histopathology, 417, 105-111.

LDL is believed to be involved in the formation of atherosclerotic plaques, and its constituent protein, apolipoprotein B, has been detected in arterial walls. Apolipoprotein (a), which associates with LDL in the circulation, has also been detected in arterial walls. This article describes an investigation into a possible correlation between immunoreactivity of apo B and apo(a) in the arterial wall. Immunohistochemical techniques were used to detect and examine the apolipoproteins in autopsy material from the left coronary artery and the thoracic aorta. The subjects were 39 females and 35 males from the ages of 0 to 98 years.

Apo(a) and apo B were found in the intima of the arterial walls in both types of arterial tissue. There was little or no staining in non-lesional areas, but a dense staining in areas with fibrous plaques and complicated lesions for both antigens, apos B and (a). The pattern of distribution of both antigens showed a high degree of congruency, suggesting that the detection of apo(a)-antigen is due in part to the presence of Lp(a), which contains apo B. The authors show that LDL and Lp(a) both have important, and possibly related, roles in the pathology of atherosclerosis.

10-22. Paulweber, B., Friedl, W., Krempler, F., Humphries, S.E., and Sandhofer, F. (1990). Association of DNA polymorphism at the apolipoprotein B gene locus with coronary heart disease and serum very low density lipoprotein levels. Arteriosclerosis, 10, 17-24.

The authors looked at genetic variability at the 3' end of the apolipoprotein B gene to see if these alleles relate to coronary heart disease.

Xba1 and EcoR1 restriction fragment length polymorphisms have been found to be associated with CHD and/or serum levels of various lipids and lipoproteins in some studies but not in others. Therefore, they examined the frequency of alleles from these two RFLPs to see if they could find an association with CHD in their Austrian population. They recruited 106 consecutive male patients with definitive coronary heart disease and 118 healthy male controls, matched for age and ethnic background. They found no difference in the allele frequency of the Xba1 polymorphism between patients and controls, but they did find a significantly higher frequency of the R2 restriction fragment of EcoR1 (24.1% of CHD patients vs. 14.4% of controls). The R2 allele was also associated with higher levels of serum triglycerides, VLDL-triglycerides, and VLDL-cholesterol. It is unlikely, however, that this allele will be useful as a marker for assessing CHD risk in the general population since it does not add to the discriminating power provided by traditional lipid parameters.

10-23. Perez, G.O., Mendez, A.J., Goldberg, R.B., Duncan, R., Palomo, A., DeMarchena, E., and Hsia, S.L. (1990). Correlates of atherosclerosis in coronary arteries of patients undergoing angiographic evaluation. Angiography, 41, 525-532.

This study evaluated the correlations between serum lipids and lipoproteins to angiographically assessed coronary heart disease. Subjects were 101 men undergoing coronary angiography to evaluate chest pain. Fasting blood was obtained for serum measurements of triglycerides, total cholesterol, and lipoprotein cholesterols by enzymatic methods. Apolipoproteins AI and B were measured by radioimmunoassay. Other risk factors such as age, obesity, smoking, family history, hypertension, and diabetes were also evaluated.

Four groups of patients were discriminated based on arteriograms: Group 1 had no detectable atherosclerotic lesions (n=24) or minimal lesions (n=2); Group 2 had single vessel disease (n=10); Group 3 had 2 vessel disease (n=22); and Group 4 had 3 vessel disease (n=43). There were no significant differences in laboratory data between patients in the three CAD groups, and, therefore, these data were combined and compared to subjects without observable coronary lesions. The two groups were significantly different in a number of respects, with the CAD patients having higher levels of serum total cholesterol, triglycerides, LDL-cholesterol, and apo B, and a higher mean age and weight. The CAD subjects also had lower levels of HDL-cholesterol, HDL_2-cholesterol, HDL_3-cholesterol, and apo AI. Despite these differences in individual measurements no single variable was able to adequately distinguish the presence or absence of atherosclerosis. Logistic regression using these data showed that 5 variables had independent predictive value: apo AI, apo B, age, diabetes, and family history of heart disease. This study confirms that apos AI and B seem to be better discriminators of CAD than traditional lipid measurements alone.

10-24. Rajput-Williams, J., Knott, T.J., Wallis, S.C., Sweetnam, P., Yarnell, J., Cox, N., Bell, G.I., Miller, N.E., and Scott, J. (1988). Variation of apolipoprotein-B gene is associated with obesity, high blood cholesterol levels, and increased risk of coronary heart disease. Lancet, 882 (8626-8627), 1442-1446.

Two-hundred-ninety males were randomly selected as part of an epidemiologic heart disease study to look for possible links between restriction fragment length polymorphisms of the apolipoprotein B gene and serum lipid levels, obesity, smoking, and coronary heart disease. An association was seen with PvuII and XbaI RFLPs and obesity, which the authors suggest is due to linkage disequilibrium of these RFLP with metabolic changes that predispose to obesity. For example, mutation of the apo B gene could affect secretion of VLDL from the liver which could lead to an increase in fat storage. MspI and EcoRI RFLPs were significantly associated with serum cholesterol levels while CHD was associated with XbaI and MspI variants. The authors summarize these results as suggesting that "inherited variations of the apolipoprotein B gene...influence circulating cholesterol concentration, and that these and other functional variants of the apolipoprotein B gene affect susceptibility to coronary heart disease and obesity." Although there appears to be a link between apo B gene variants and plasma cholesterol levels and obesity, the authors may not be justified in relating RFLPs to heart disease risk based on these data.

10-25. Rath, M., Niendorf, A., Reblin, T., Dietel, M., Krebber, H.-J., and Beisiegel, U. (1989). Detection and quantification of lipoprotein (a) in the arterial wall of 107 coronary bypass patients. Arteriosclerosis, 9, 579-592.

This study looked at lipoprotein (a) accumulation in the arterial wall in relation to serum Lp(a) concentration and its potential role in atherosclerosis. Blood was collected preoperatively from 306 patients (250 men, 56 women, mean age 57 years) undergoing coronary bypass surgery. Twenty percent of the patients were taking lipid lowering medications but only 3% had normal lipid values. Control subjects (n=72) were matched for age and sex. Tissue biopsies were obtained from 107 of the bypass patients for histological exam. Lipoprotein fractions were separated by density gradient ultracentrifugation. Lp(a) in serum and tissue was measured by radial immunodiffusion; tissue apo(a) and plasma apos B and (a) were measured by ELISA and by radioimmunoassay. Post mortem biopsy samples were collected from the aorta and main stem of the left coronary artery of 11 individuals for immunohistochemical analysis.

There were significant differences between the patient and control groups; the CHD group had higher levels of total cholesterol, triglycerides, and VLDL-cholesterol, and lower HDL-cholesterol concentrations. CHD patients also had a much higher mean serum Lp(a) level (25 vs 14 mg/dl) while 40% of the patients and only 16% of the controls had Lp(a) concentrations over 25 mg/dl. There was a significant correlation between apo(a) and apo(a)-linked apo B in aortic biopsy samples with serum levels of Lp(a); however, the amount of apo(a)-B complex varied widely. No significant correlation was seen between serum apo B and arterial wall apo B. Also, the apo(a) isoform distribution in this tissue was the same as the plasma apo(a) isoform pattern. The post mortem arterial wall samples were divided into two groups based on the amount of plaque, < or > 50%. There was no difference between these two groups with respect to total tissue triglycerides or total protein, but the samples with > 50% plaque area had higher concentrations of cholesterol, apo B, and apo(a). As expected, apo B and apo(a) were found in the intima, and the distribution of these proteins were similar, suggesting that Lp(a) is involved in the atherosclerotic process.

In summary, this is a detailed study which provides evidence for Lp(a) involvement in plaque formation and coronary artery disease progression.

10-26. Reinhart, R.A., Gani, K., Arndt, M.R., and Broste, S.K. (1990). Apolipoproteins A-I and B as predictors of angiographically defined coronary artery disease. Archives of Internal Medicine, 150, 1629-1633.

In this study apolipoproteins AI and B were determined in 502 patients, including 154 women, undergoing cardiac catheterization to angiographically assess coronary artery disease. They compared the predictive power of these apolipoprotein levels to the strength of association of traditional CAD risk factors such as serum cholesterol level. Serum was analyzed for total cholesterol, LDL-cholesterol, HDL-cholesterol, triglycerides, apo AI, and apo B concentrations. Angiograms were graded as normal, mild, moderate, or severe. Controls were those subjects whose angiograms proved negative.

The authors found no significant difference in apo AI concentration between normal subjects and subjects with any degree of CAD in either men or women, but apo B and the apo AI/apo B ratio were significantly different between cases and controls in both sexes. Total cholesterol, LDL-cholesterol, and non-HDL-cholesterol were also different between cases and controls in men. Among the women, the mean values for the HDL-cholesterol/total cholesterol ratio and triglycerides were the only lipids showing a significant difference. Based on two logistic regression models, one based on standard lipid values and one based on apolipoproteins, the authors conclude that the model with apolipoprotein measures provided more accurate classification than the standard lipid measures.

In summary, this article demonstrates the value of apo B and the apo AI/apo B ratio, in addition to traditional lipid measurements, in predicting the presence of CAD. As the authors point out, their control population was not carefully selected. They selected a group that contained a high proportion of patients with CAD, and the controls were patients who were being examined for possible CAD but whose angiograms proved negative; so they were not necessarily healthy controls. Also, since these patients had previous histories of cardiovascular disease, they may have been counselled to modify their diet or lifestyle which would minimize differences between the two groups.

10-27. Ronnemaa, T., Laakso, M., Kallio, V., Pyorala, K., Marniemi, J., and Puukka, P. (1989). Serum lipids, lipoproteins, and apolipoproteins and the excessive occurrence of coronary heart disease in non-insulin-dependent diabetic patients. American Journal of Epidemiology, 130, 632-645.

This was a very ambitious study involving many different parameters. The authors proposed to answer the following questions:

(1)   Is the atherogenic pattern of lipids and lipoproteins seen   in diabetics a reflection of the disease itself or is it secondary to other confounding variables such as obesity,

(2)   Are the same associations of lipid parameters seen in heart disease patients similar to heart disease in diabetic patients, and

(3)   Are these associations of lipid parameters similar in diabetics and non-diabetics from East and West Finland; areas that are different with respect to the incidence of heart disease.

More than 500 diabetics, 253 men and 257 women, were recruited from East Finland; and 549 diabetics, 328 men and 221 women, were recruited from West Finland. Nondiabetic subjects of the same age range and geographic distribution were randomly selected as controls. Myocardial infarct patients were identified by electrocardiogram and from medical records. Serum was measured for total cholesterol, triglycerides, HDL-cholesterol, apo AI (by radioimmunoassay), and apo B (by immunoturbidimetry).

Diabetic patients had higher serum triglycerides, apo B, and a higher apo B/apo A ratio. With some exceptions, these differences persisted after adjusting for body mass index, alcohol intake, physical activity, smoking, and hypertension. The associations of these lipid, lipoprotein, and apolipoproteins were similar in both groups of MI patients, diabetic or nondiabetic. These associations were also the same between East and West Findlanders. There are many interesting observations described in this paper, such as the association of serum triglycerides with a low HDL-cholesterol/apo AI ratio. This may indicate that a high level of triglycerides decreases the cholesterol transporting ability of the HDL-particle while not affecting the metabolism of apo AI.

In general, this is a well-controlled study showing that heart disease associated with non-insulin dependent diabetes mellitus is inherent in the disease itself and is not simply secondary to other risk factors. In addition, this article sheds light on other areas of lipid metabolism such as the interrelationship of serum triglycerides and HDL-cholesterol metabolism.

10-28. Sandkamp, M., Funke, H., Schulte, H., Kohler, E., and Assman, G. (1990). Lipoprotein (a) is an independent risk factor for myocardial infarction at a young age. Clinical Chemistry, 36 (1), 20-23.

This article describes a very ambitious investigation of Lp(a) concentration in relation to other well known risk factors for heart disease. Subjects were myocardial infarction survivors; 509 males less than 46 years old and 1053 age-matched control subjects selected from the Prospective Cardiovascular Munster Study. Apos AI, AII, B, and Lp(a) levels, and apo E polymorphisms were determined, along with total serum cholesterol, HDL-cholesterol, serum triglycerides, and LDL-cholesterol.

Cardiac patients had significantly higher levels of total cholesterol, apo B, and Lp(a), and significantly lower levels of HDL-cholesterol, apo AI, and apo AII. The mean value of Lp(a) for MI survivors was 0.12 vs 0.05 g/L for controls. They found no correlation between Lp(a) and LDL-cholesterol in controls or patients, nor between apo E phenotype and Lp(a). There was also a lack of association between age and Lp(a) levels. This was a very thorough study clearly showing Lp(a) to be an independent risk factor for heart disease.

10-29. Seed, M., Hoppichler, F., Reaveley, D., McCarthy, S., Thompson, G.R., Boerwinkle, E., and Utermann, G. (1990). Relation of serum lipoprotein (a) concentration and apolipoprotein (a) phenotype to coronary heart disease in patients with hypercholesterolemia. New England Journal of Medicine, 322, 1494-1499.

The authors point out that individuals with familial hypercholesterolemia have an increased risk of coronary heart disease, but there is considerable variation among individuals with this disorder in susceptibility to CHD. Therefore, they investigated lipoprotein (a) association with CHD in 115 patients with heterozygous familial hypercholesterolemia. Sixty-one men and 54 women were selected from among patients at a London hospital lipid clinic; all were white and at least 20 years old. The group was further classified based on a diagnosis of CHD as assessed by a history of angina, positive exercise test, abnormal coronary angiogram (>70% stenosis of a major vessel), or a history of previous myocardial infarction.

Among the CHD group there were significantly more smokers and they had a significantly higher mean age, but there was no difference in the proportion of individuals who were hypertensive. Also, there were no differences in serum total cholesterol, LDL-cholesterol, or HDL-cholesterol levels. Serum triglyceride level was higher in the CHD group as was median Lp(a) concentration (57 vs 18 mg/dl). There was no correlation between Lp(a) levels and age or sex. Stepwise multiple discriminant analysis found Lp(a) to be the best discriminator between the two groups. The investigators also compared apo(a) phenotypes and found a higher frequency of the Lp^{s1} and Lp^{s2} alleles and a lower frequency of the Lp^{s4} allele among CHD patients. However, adding apo(a) phenotypes to their predictive equation, which included Lp(a) concentration, did not contribute further in assessing CHD risk. This research shows rather conclusively that Lp(a) is a strong, independent risk factor for CHD in patients with familial hypercholesterolemia.

10-30.   Stampfer, M.J., Sacks, F.M., Salvini, S., Willett, W.C., and Hennekens, C.H. (1991). A prospective study of cholesterol, apolipoproteins, and the risk of myocardial infarction. New England Journal of Medicine, 325, 373-381.

This article is the only large, comprehensive, prospective study of apolipoproteins in relation to cardiovascular disease of which I am aware. Subjects were participants in the Physicians' Health Study, an ongoing randomized, double-blind, placebo-controlled trial of aspirin and beta-carotene. Individuals who had suffered an MI during the five year follow-up period (n=246) were matched for age and smoking status with 246 control subjects. Lipids were measured enzymatically, and apolipoproteins were measured by radial immunodiffusion.

Subjects with previous MI had a higher BMI, blood pressure, prevalence of angina and diabetes, and increased plasma levels of total cholesterol and total cholesterol/HDL-cholesterol ratio. Subjects with MI also had decreased levels of HDL-cholesterol, HDL_2-cholesterol, HDL_3-cholesterol, apo AI, and HDL particles without apo AII. Conditional logistic regression showed increased relative risk of MI with increasing levels of total cholesterol and apo B, and decreasing risk with increasing levels of HDL-cholesterol, HDL subfraction-cholesterol, apo AI, and HDL particles without apo AII. Total cholesterol/HDL-cholesterol ratio was the most powerful predictor of risk, with the risk of MI almost four times greater for individuals in the highest quintile compared with individuals in the lowest quintile. The authors found no evidence that adding levels of apolipoproteins to a multivariate model that included the ratio of total cholesterol to HDL-cholesterol and non-lipid risk factors added any predictive value, despite the fact that apos AI, AII, and B were all significant predictors of risk individually.

These conclusions differ sharply with the results of other studies. This study has the advantage of a prospective design, but there is room for criticism. Although it was not included in the authors' regression equation, elevated LDL-cholesterol is an established cardiovascular disease risk factor. Because LDL-cholesterol was not measured in this study the predictive value of apo B and LDL-cholesterol could not be compared. Therefore, I do not think the authors are completely justified in rejecting the value of apo B measurement. Secondly, the subjects of this study are not representative of the general population. As the authors point out, "participants in the Physicians' Health Study are unusually healthy, with cardiovascular mortality only 15% that of the general population of white men of comparable age in the United States." I do not think that this study is conclusive simply because it is prospective. Clearly, more prospective data are needed.

10-31. Tasaki, H., Nakashima, Y., Nandate, H., Yashiro, A., Kawashima, T., and Kuroiwa, A. (1989). Comparison of serum lipid values in variant angina pectoris and fixed coronary artery disease with normal subjects. <u>American Journal of Cardiology</u>, <u>63</u>, 1441-1445.

This study compared plasma lipids and apolipoprotein concentrations in control subjects and patients with two forms of coronary artery disease, variant angina pectoris and fixed coronary artery disease. Male patients, aged 30 to 74 years, undergoing coronary angiography were classified according to diagnosis and degree of stenosis. Seventy-eight subjects had either variant angina or fixed CAD and significant atherosclerotic lesions (> 50% stenosis). The remaining 30 subjects comprised the control group. Blood was collected for enzymatic measurement of plasma and lipoprotein cholesterol and triglyceride content. Apolipoproteins AI, AII, B, CII, CIII, and apo E were measured by radioimmunodiffusion.

Apo AI levels in variant angina and fixed CAD patients were significantly lower than in the control group, and only apo AI was able to discriminate among the three groups. As the authors point out, the percent accuracy in classifying these subject was too small to be clinically useful.

10-32. Thieszen, S.L., Hixson, J.E., Nagengast, D.J., Wilson, J.E., and McManus, B.M. (1990). Lipid phenotypes, apolipoprotein genotypes and cardiovascular risk in nonagenarians. <u>Atherosclerosis, 83</u>, 137-146.

These authors are interested in identifying factors which may contribute to longevity; especially factors which relate to a reduced risk for atherosclerosis.

Thirty-one females and 10 males from rural Nebraska, over age 90, were recruited as subjects. Data were collected for 24-hour food intake, exercise, smoking, alcohol consumption, blood pressure, height, weight, triceps skinfold thickness, serum total cholesterol, lipoprotein cholesterols, and apolipoproteins AI and B. Cholesterol was measured enzymatically by a commercial laboratory; apos AI and B were measured by immunonephelometry. Additionally, blood from 23 subjects was used for RFLP analysis with three restriction enzymes.

Most subjects responded that they had never consumed alcohol, had never used tobacco, and exercised regularly. Diastolic blood pressures were all normal and only two subjects had a systolic blood pressure greater than 150 mm Hg. Subjects with BMI values below the mean (25.2 for males and 23.4 for females) had significantly lower LDL-cholesterol levels and significantly lower skinfold thicknesses. Total cholesterol, HDL-cholesterol, and the LDL-cholesterol/apo B ratio also tended to be different based on this BMI division. Of the 26 nursing home residents, 21 were diagnosed with coronary heart disease and most were taking a variety of medications. It would have been interesting to know more specifically how these parameters related to the overall health of these individuals; perhaps the healthier subjects had lower BMIs and LDL cholesterols, for example. The diets of these subjects tended to be higher in carbohydrates, while caloric intakes varied considerably. Similarly, lipid levels were very diverse. RFLPs at four restriction sites; two at the apo AI gene, one at the apo CIII gene, and one at the apo B gene, indicate that nonagenarians are not distinguished by any particular allelic frequency. As the authors suggest, the lack of any consistent data provides insight into the complexity of longevity.

10-33. Wile, D.B., Barbir, M., Gallagher, J., Myant, N.B., Ritchie, C.D., Thompson, G.R., and Humphries, S. E. (1989). Apolipoprotein A-I gene polymorphisms: Frequencies in patients with coronary artery disease and healthy controls and association with serum Apo A-I and HDL-cholesterol concentration. Atherosclerosis, 78, 9-18.

The authors investigated restriction fragment length polymorphisms of the apo AI gene and their possible association with serum HDL-cholesterol and apo AI concentrations. Male patients with angiographic evidence of coronary artery disease (n=174) were compared to 104 healthy males. Serum total cholesterol, triglycerides, HDL-cholesterol, apo B, and apo AI were measured; apo B was determined by radial immunodiffusion and apo AI was measured by an immunoturbidimetric technique. DNA was digested with the restriction enzymes XmnI and PstI.

The PstI enzyme produces a fragment due to an allele which is designated P2. P2 was twice as common in CAD patients compared to control subjects. There were no differences in allele frequencies of the XmnI polymorphism between patients and controls. CAD patients with the P1P2 genotype from the PstI enzyme cut had a mean HDL-cholesterol and apo AI level lower than individuals with the P1P1 genotype. For the control group, however, there was no difference in HDL-cholesterol, but subjects with the P1P2 genotype had a higher AI concentration compared to P1P1 individuals. Patients with the X1X2 genotype of the XmnI polymorphism had an average apo AI and HDL-cholesterol level significantly higher than individuals with the X1X1 genotype, while in controls there were no significant differences.

These data show that PstI polymorphism is associated with a predisposition to CAD. This is contradictory to two previous studies, which again illustrates the ambiguity often seen with RFLP techniques.

10-34. Wilson, H.M., Patel, J.C., and Skinner, E.R. (1990). Plasma high-density lipoprotein subfractions in survivors of myocardial infarction. Biochemical Society Transactions, 18, 330.

HDL has been shown to be protective against coronary heart disease. It has further been demonstrated that the protective effect is due predominantly to the larger HDL particles. HDL particles also contain different apolipoproteins which may differentiate protective HDL from neutral HDL. Apo E, for example, is thought by many to be involved in the efflux of cholesterol from the arterial wall by HDL. In this study blood was collected from 88 males, aged 40-65 years, who had previously had a myocardial infarction. VLDL, LDL, and HDL were separated by ultracentrifugation, and HDL was further separated by gradient gel electrophoresis and quantitated using densitometry. Apo E-containing HDL was separated by heparin-sepharose affinity chromatography.

The mean concentrations of cholesterol in HDL, HDL_2, HDL_3, HDL_{2b}, and apo E-rich HDL were all lower in the plasmas of the coronary patients than in healthy subjects, while total plasma cholesterol and LDL-cholesterol were not significantly different between the 2 groups. The authors did find a strong negative correlation between the smallest particle, HDL_{3c}, and the larger particles, HDL_{3a} and HDL_{2a}, in heart disease patients, which suggests an impaired conversion of the smaller, newly synthesized particles into mature particles which can carry more cholesterol. Unfortunately, this is only a preliminary study and much of the data were not presented, but it is an important observation that interconversion of HDL particles may be important in the development of atherosclerosis.

11

GROWTH HORMONE
AND AGING

John Contois

INTRODUCTION

A recent study in the New England Journal of Medicine describing the effects of growth hormone (GH) administration in the elderly received considerable media attention. Amazing anti-aging effects were described, including improved muscle strength, healthier skin, increased muscle mass, loss of adipose tissue, and improved vigor. Newspaper reports stated that participants looked and acted "20 years younger," and that "the effects of six months of GH on lean body mass and adipose tissue were equivalent in magnitude to the changes incurred during 10-20 years of aging." This study (Rudman et al., NEJM, 1990, 323, 1-6) was a long term, comprehensive study with promising results, but the media perception that this is a "fountain of youth" is unwarranted.

Growth hormone was isolated about 30 years ago when it was found to be necessary for linear growth in children. More recently, it has been found to be important for many normal anabolic processes throughout the lifespan. The recent studies with exogenous GH have become possible with the production of human GH by recombinant DNA techniques. The anabolic effects of GH are due to the direct action of the hormone itself and via its stimulation of insulin-like growth factor I (IGF-I, also called somatomedin C). In the articles I have summarized, it is demonstrated that the physiology of these two hormones is intimately linked. In terms of development, GH secretion increases dramatically at puberty, then decreases in late adolescence, and remains stable until approximately age 30. After age 30 GH decreases progressively into the later years. Diurnally, GH is stimulated episodically and is, therefore, measured at a number of different time points in most studies.

This brief review of the literature asks two questions. First, is GH deficiency common in the elderly and is this decline related to physiological changes? Second, what are the benefits and risks of GH replacement therapy in older adults?

It is clear from this literature that most elderly secrete much less GH than younger adults, and this decline correlates with an increase in adiposity and a loss in lean body mass. The study of Rudman et al., 1981, is noteworthy because it demonstrates a progressive decline in GH levels with each decade of life. In an interesting study Kelly et al. show that some anabolic effects of GH and IGF-I may be due to the improved fitness which is associated with higher levels of these hormones and not the direct action of the hormones themselves.

With the availability of human GH for replacement therapy the question of causality can be directly assessed. In the few studies that have been done GH administration has resulted in an increase in lean body mass and a decrease in adipose tissue mass. In the shorter term studies in which nitrogen balance was used to estimate anabolic responsiveness, GH administration did result in increased nitrogen retention. All four studies in the elderly show positive anabolic effects of exogenous GH. In the most thorough study to date Rudman et al., 1990, report improvements in IGF-I concentration, lean body mass, bone density, skin thickness, and a decrease in body fat. The only side effects were a slight but significant increase in the mean systolic blood pressure and an increase in fasting serum glucose. Whether or not these changes are important clinically is not discussed.

The other intervention studies are all short term and all report increases in IGF-I and nitrogen retention. Marcus et al. report an increase in anabolic parameters associated with bone formation. Unfortunately, it is hard to interpret the data because the positive changes in vitamin D, PTH, osteocalcin, etc, may simply be a response to the increased calcium excretion in urine. Binnerts et al. also report a negative calcium balance with GH treatment, although this may be the result of a very high protein diet. Clearly this ambiguity regarding GH effects on bone metabolism is the only negative outcome from these data. GH has a clear anabolic effect even at low physiologic doses, and the side effects, other than the effects on calcium and bone, do not appear to be clinically important.

ANNOTATED BIBLIOGRAPHY

11-1. Binnerts, A., Wilson, J.H.P., and Lamberts, S.W.J. (1988). The effects of human growth hormone administration in elderly adults with recent weight loss. Journal of Clinical Endocrinology and Metabolism, 67, 1312-1316.

In this study low doses of GH were administered to underweight elderly given optimal nutritional support to see if this treatment could induce nitrogen retention without causing important changes in glucose tolerance or fluid balance. The subjects were two men, aged 59 and 70 years, and two women aged 51 and 80 years. These patients required enteral nutritional support for weight loss due to non-malignant illness. They did not have metabolic disorders such as renal or hepatic disease or diabetes, but one patient did have a hypopituitary disorder and was GH deficient. The subjects were admitted to a metabolic study ward for a period of 24 days and given an enteral, mixed diet containing 120% or more of the recommended energy and protein requirements based on age and size. After a 3-day period to acheive metabolic balance the experimental period began. On days 5-8 the subjects received 25 ug GH/kg body weight per day subcutaneously at 9:00 AM. On days 13-16 the dose was increased to 50 ug/kg body weight per day.

GH was well tolerated by all four patients. There were no changes in kidney or liver function tests, electrolytes, cholesterol or triglycerides, total protein, albumin, or leukocyte count. Nitrogen retention significantly increased during the GH administration phases in all 4 subjects, and the effect was prolonged at the higher dose. Plasma IGF-I rose during both periods of GH administration from subnormal to high normal values. Body weight increased during both GH treatment phases also, but decreased within days when treatment ended. The mean maximal increase in body weight, 2.3 ± 0.6 kg, was postulated to be an increase in fluid retention, although they do not explain why. GH treatment was also associated with a negative calcium balance.

In summary, this study shows that GH can increase nitrogen retention in underweight elderly, even while receiving adequate nutritional support. However, these subjects were ill and the authors fail to describe what effects GH may have had in improving their overall health. In fact, the treatment may have even worsened the patients' condition by increasing urinary calcium loss. Since only four subjects were described in this study it would have been interesting for the authors to include more descriptive and less structured data and information.

11-2. Degerblad, M., Grunditz, R., Hall, K., Sjoberg, H.E., Saaf, M., and Thoren, M. (1987). Substitution therapy with recombinant growth hormone (Somatrem) in adults with growth hormone deficiency. <u>Acta Paediatr Scand</u> [Supplement], <u>337</u>, 170-171.

This report briefly describes the results of a pilot study in which the effects of GH therapy were evaluated over a 12-week period. The parameters investigated included physical capacity, muscle strength, bone mineral content, cognitive function, and mood. The subjects were three women and three men aged 20-30 years with GH deficiency. The symptoms of GH deficiency in these subjects were general fatigue, low physical capacity, and poor muscle strength; one subject was hypoglycemic. In a double-blind crossover design GH or placebo was administered for 12 weeks with a 12 week washout period in between. GH was administered at a dose of 4 IU subcutaneously, six or seven nights per week. Psychological tests for cognitive function and mood were also performed.

In the initial screening the physical exercise test was normal for four of the six subjects, and bone mineral content was low in all six subjects. After the study was completed five of the six subjects could correctly identify their treatment period with GH, and the authors reported "positive subjective effects...generally improved well-being...increased mental alertness, increased work capacity and improved muscle strength." However, the data did not show any significant differences in the physical exercise test, dynamic muscle strength, or bone mineral content between the placebo and treatment periods. There was, however, an increase in procollagen III peptide and serum IGF-I and a decrease in serum urea in the treatment phase. Self rated mood scales showed a tendency for improvement of symptoms of depression and cognitive tests showed improved verbal learning with GH treatment.

This is an interesting paper because it assesses cognitive function, mood and self-reported perceptions of well-being as well as the traditional physiologic parameters. This proves to be important since physiologic parameters changed very little if at all, yet treatment appears to improve the patients' feeling of wellness and mood. Perhaps the techniques used were not sensitive enough to detect any improvements with the GH therapy or perhaps the treatment was not long enough to induce these changes. However, this was only a pilot study. It is an interesting approach that shows the value of subjective and self-reported subject data in a discipline that does not usually value such data.

11-3.   Finkelstein, J.W., Roffwarg, H.P., Boyar, R.M., Kream, J., and Hellman, L. (1972). Age related change in the twenty four hour spontaneous secretion of growth hormone. Journal of Clinical Endocrinology and Metabolism, 35, 665-670.

This study demonstrated an age-associated alteration in the 24-hour pattern of spontaneous GH secretion in plasma. The subjects were four prepubertal boys 8-15 years old, four boys and six girls 9-20 years old, in various stages of development, and five women and four men aged 23-62. All subjects were healthy and not taking any medications. The study was conducted in a clinical research ward. On the first night subjects were adapted to the sleep study procedure and monitored to precisely identify sleep stages. Starting the next morning an indwelling catheter was inserted to allow for the sequential collection of blood for growth hormone analysis. A rise of 5 ng/ml was considered to be a secretory episode.

For prepubertal children GH was secreted only during sleep. During waking hours there were not any significant secretory peaks. Total secretion during a 24-hour period was 54-122 ug with a mean of 91 ug. There were only 1-3 secretory episodes per subject. Adolescents secreted GH during wakefulness and sleep with 1-4 episodes during the day and another 1-4 episodes during sleep. A mean of 230 ug was secreted during wakefulness and a mean of 460 ug was secreted during sleep; significantly more than in prepuberty. Young adults aged 23-42 also secreted GH during wakefulness (six of eight individuals) at an average of 141 ug. During sleep GH was secreted in 1 or 2 episodes averaging 241 ug (significantly different from both previous groups). Older adults, aged 47- 52 had no detectable secretion of GH in three of the five individuals studied. One individual had only one secretory period during wakefulness and none at night, while another individual had no detectable amounts of GH at all.

These data clearly show an age-related change in the spontaneous 24-hour secretion of GH with the oldest individuals secreting the least amount of GH.

11-4. Florini, J.R., Prinz, P.N., Vitiello, M.V., and Hintz, R.L. (1985). Somatomedin-C Levels in healthy young and old men: Relationship to peak and 24-hour integrated levels of growth hormone. Journal of Gerontology, 40, 2-7.

The authors believe that many reports on the association between somatomedin-C (Sm-C) and GH are flawed because the diurnal fluctuations in GH levels and its short half-life are not taken into account. A single measurement may not reflect the true physiology of the hormone. Also, measurement of both hormones, but especially Sm-C, are uncertain because binding proteins can mask the true concentration of the hormone. To clarify the relationship between GH and Sm-C, levels of these hormones were determined in younger and older men at different time points across a 24-hour period. The subjects were paid volunteers, 17 aged 23-27 years and 13 aged 58-82 years; all were normotensive, nonobese, nonsmokers, in good physical health as assessed by a physical exam, medical history, and electrocardiogram. They were studied in a controlled metabolic study ward and given a standard hospital diet. For the first day the subjects were given time to adapt to the surroundings; the second day was for data and sample collection. Indwelling catheters were inserted for regular blood drawing; blood sampled from three representative times were assayed for Sm-C after running the sample through an acidified column to separate Sm-C activity from binding protein.

For Sm-C a significant age effect was seen with no significant time or interaction effects. In other words, Sm-C levels are not subject to diurnal variation despite the wide fluctuations in GH levels. The mean Sm-C concentrations were 0.95 and 0.68 U/ml for young and old men, respectively, and mean Sm-C level was significantly correlated with the 24-hour integrated

GH level in plasma. There was not, however, any correlation of Sm-C with any single episode of GH secretion. The significant correlation between Sm-C and 24-hour integrated GH levels for the combined young and old adults suggests that the age related decline in Sm-C levels is the direct result of a decrease in GH secretion by the pituitary. This decrease could be an important determinant in the age related changes in bone and muscle.

The authors' description of the experimental design is not clear in terms of what data were collected in each individual or what time points were used for hormone determinations. Still the data clarify the relationship between GH and Sm-C and suggests that Sm-C is an intermediate in the effect of GH on muscle and bone metabolism.

11-5.   Ho, K.Y., Evans, W.S., Blizzard, R.M., Veldhuis, J.D., Merriam, G.R., Samojlik, E., Furlanetto, R., Rogol, A.D., Kaiser, D.L., and Thorner, M.O. (1987). Effects of sex and age on the 24-hour profile of growth hormone secretion in man: Importance of endogenous estradiol concentrations. Journal of Clinical Endocrinology and Metabolism, 64, 51-58.

This study examined age and sex differences in GH secretion over a 24-hour period. The authors believe that differences between studies may be due to differences in the subjects; that is, age and sex differences. In this study subjects were 10 young women, 18-33 years old; 10 young men, aged 18-30 years; eight post-menopausal women, 57-76 years old; and eight older men, aged 56-71 years. The subjects were in good health and eating their regular diets when admitted for the overnight study. They were admitted in the morning after an overnight fast, and had an intravenous catheter inserted for blood drawing at regular intervals. Twenty-four hour GH profile was assessed in terms of total secretion (integrated GH concentration, IGHC), the fraction of total GH secreted as pulses (FGHP), and pulse frequency, magnitude, and duration.

IGHC, FGHP, GH pulse magnitude and duration, and number of GH pulses were all significantly lower in the older subjects. Age related changes in GH secretion occured primarily in women, and sex related differences occured primarily between younger individuals. The data also show a strong correlation between estradiol concentration and GH, and that the effects of age and sex on IGHC secretion are not independent of the effects of estradiol, although the authors concede that "aging still had a significant effect on the residual variability."

The authors try to minimize the importance of aging as an independent cause of declining GH secretion. They show conclusively that estrogens correlate with GH concentrations and age, but they cannot account for all of the variability in GH levels. Their data show that there is a greater change in GH parameters in women with aging, for example, that is statistically stronger than the change in men, but there is clearly a change in men as well that may be physiologically important, if not statistically important. Still, the observation of an association between GH and estrogen is important.

11-6. Kelly, P.J., Eisman, J.A., Stuart, M.C., Pocock, N.A., Sambrook, P.N., and Gwinn, T.H. (1990). Somatomedin-C, physical fitness, and bone density. Journal of Clinical Endocrinology and Metabolism, 70, 718-723.

The objective of this study was to see if the age related change in circulating levels of GH and Sm-C may be related to an age related decline in physical fitness and muscle strength, and secondly, to see if the effect of physical fitness and muscle strength on bone may be mediated by Sm-C. The subjects were 177 female volunteers with a mean age of 46 years and a range from 19 to 83; 69 were post menopausal. Mean body mass index was 23.7 kg/m^2. Subjects had no previous history of bone disease, illness or drug use which would affect bone density, and none had impaired renal function. The data show a positive correlation between VO_2 max (an estimate of physical fitness) and both GH and Sm-C. Plasma Sm-C correlated with GH as well, and both GH and Sm-C declined with increasing age. Both VO_2 max and overall muscle strength correlated with age, and overall muscle strength correlated with GH level but not Sm-C concentration. Backward elimination multiple regression analysis was used to examine the interrelationship between Sm-C and the other variables: age, BMI, VO_2 max, GH, estradiol, and menopausal state. VO_2 max was the only significant independent predictor of plasma Sm-C and plasma GH concentrations. Excluding $VO_{2\,max,}$ age was the only independent predictor of GH level.

In summary, the authors show that Sm-C and GH levels are related to VO2 max in normal females. Secondly, they confirm the findings of an inverse relationship between both Sm-C and GH and age; however, this relationship may not be independent of other variables, such as fitness. This is the first report of a relationship between physical fitness and plasma levels of GH and Sm-C. As a correlational study it points out the complex interactions between variables that need to be further investigated.

11-7. Marcus, R., Butterfield, G., Holloway, L., Gilliland, L., Baylink, D.J., Hintz, R.L., and Sherman, B.M. (1990). Effects of short term administration of recombinant human growth hormone to elderly people. Journal of Clinical Epidemiology and Metabolism, 70, 519-527.

The purpose of this study was to see if GH administration would substantially improve nitrogen conservation, muscle strength, and bone mass without serious side effects. The subjects were 12 women and six men, 60 years of age or older, recruited from the community. The screening procedure included a health history questionaire, physical exam, nutritional assessment, electrocardiogram, chest x-ray, urinalysis, and lab profile. The subjects chosen were in good health and were not glucose intolerant as assessed by a 2-hour postprandial plasma glucose concentration less than 120 mg/dl. A comparison group was made up of six healthy men less than 33 years old. Prior to the 12-day protocol was a 6-day dietary stabilization period. The diet was formulated to provide 1 gram of protein/kg ideal body weight per day. After the dietary stabilization period the subjects were admitted to the Aging Study Unit at Stanford University for the 12-day nitrogen balance study. On the third night an indwelling cannula was established to collect blood every 30 minutes for GH and IGF-I determinations. Human GH was given every morning at 8:00 AM from days 4 to 10 by subcutaneous injection; the subjects were randomly assigned to one of three dosage levels: 0.03, 0.06, or 0.12 mg/kg body weight.

All subjects tolerated the GH treatment. There were no significant changes in weight or blood pressure, but hematocrit and hemoglobin levels were significantly decreased. The authors attribute this to the loss of approximately 800 ml of blood over the 12-day period. They do not speculate on whether or not this may have influenced their data, but this could certainly affect some metabolic processes, including the conservation of nitrogen. The mean fasting GH concentration was 0.61 ug/L for the entire group, and was not different between men and women. The mean fasting IGF-I and GH concentrations at the beginning of the study were slightly lower in the study group than in younger controls. IGF-I concentrations increased substantially after treatment with GH. Many subjects showed mildly impaired glucose tolerance with GH treatment, although fasting glucose values were normal. This was mostly observed with the highest dose of GH, however. There were also significant reductions in total plasma cholesterol with all doses of GH. There were no changes in renal function as assessed by creatinine clearance, but the 24-hour excretion of total and urea nitrogen was significantly reduced. For the entire group 24-hour nitrogen excretion decreased from a mean of 8.0 to a mean of 5.0 g. Sodium excretion also decreased, serum inorganic phosphorus increased, serum PTH increased, serum vitamin D increased, and serum osteocalcin increased. Serum calcium levels did not change, but urinary calcium excretion increased with all doses of GH.

In summary, these results confirm that older adults have decreased overnight circulating levels of GH and IGF-I compared to younger adults, but older adults still respond to exogenous GH treatment as evidenced by a rapid increase in IGF-I and positive nitrogen balance. Unfortunately, the changes observed in nitrogen balance can be partly explained by the large blood loss leading to an increase in anabolic processes. Also, the results from data on proteins and hormones involved in bone metabolism (vitamin D, PTH, osteocalcin, etc.) can be partly explained as a response to the increased calcium loss in the urine, not as a direct response to GH.

11-8. Rudman, D., Feller, A.G., Nagraj, H.S., Gergans, G.A., LaLitha, P.Y., Goldberg, A.F., Schlenker, R.A., Cohn, L., Rudman, I.W., and Mattson, D.E. (1990). Effects of human growth hormone in men over 60 years old. New England Journal of Medicine, 323, 1-6.

The purpose of this study was to test whether or not the reduction in the activities of GH and IGF-I with advancing age is contributing to the change in body composition that occurs with aging. The subjects were 21 healthy men, aged 61-81 years old, with plasma IGF-I concentrations less than 350 U/L. Additionally, their body weights were within 90-120% of the standard for age, they had no signs of underlying disease, and they had to have the ability to administer the growth hormone to themselves by injection, subcutaneously. The screening included a physical exam, medical history, complete blood count, urinalysis, blood chemistry tests, chest x-ray, and electrocardiogram.

The protocol was 12 months long with a baseline period of six months. During this initial period the men were examined at regular intervals, and then randomly assigned to either the treatment group (n=12) or the control group (n=9). The treatment group was instructed to administer a dose of GH (0.03 mg/kg body weight) 3 times per week at 8:00 AM. Blood was collected each month 24 hours after an injection, and in some instances the dose was adjusted to keep IGF-I in the normal range. The control group received no injections. The diet throughout the 12 month protocol was planned to provide 15% of calories as protein, 50% as carbohydrate, and 35% as fat.

Their results were as follows. No individual experienced any changes in differential blood count, urinalysis, blood chemistry profile, chest radiography, electrocardiogram; none had edema, fasting hyperglycemia, ventricular hypertrophy, or any reaction or side effects to the GH treatment. In the treatment group mean systolic blood pressure and fasting glucose increased significantly at the end of the treatment period, but the change was not considered clinically important. Mean plasma IGF-I ranged from 200-250 U/L throughout the baseline period, but increased to a mean of 830 U/L within one month of treatment. There was no significant change in body weight in either group, but lean body mass increased 8.8 %, bone density of the lumbar vertebrae increased 1.6%, adipose tissue mass decreased 14.4%, and skin thickness increased 7.1% in the treatment group compared with controls.

In conclusion, in men with low plasma IGF-I concentrations, responsiveness to GH treatment was not impaired. Therefore, the decrease in plasma IGF-I probably results from GH deficiency and not resistance. Secondly, these findings confirm the hypothesis that the decrease in lean body mass and increase in adipose tissue, as well as skin changes that occur with aging, are due, at least in part, to reduced activity of GH and IGF-I. Finally, these data show that replacement therapy with GH at physiological levels restores the beneficial effects of these hormones.

11-9.   Rudman, D., Kutner, M.H., Rogers, C.M., Lubin, M.F., Fleming, G.A., and Bain, R.P. (1981). Impaired growth hormone secretion in the adult population: Relation to age and adiposity. Journal of Clinical Investigation, 67, 1361-1369.

This was perhaps the first intervention study administering human growth hormone (GH) to adults. The purpose of this study was to investigate the prevalence of impaired GH secretion in adults by measuring endogenous GH secretion and plasma Sm-C levels at various time points, and also to see if anabolic processes respond to exogenous GH administration. The subjects were 72 individuals from age 21-86 years who met the following criteria: 85-115% of ideal body weight, 5-95th percentile for height, no detectable disease, resting systolic blood pressure < 160 mm Hg, diastolic BP < 90 mm Hg: urinalysis, urine culture, hematocrit, blood urea nitrogen, serum creatinine, serum albumin, fasting and 2-hour post-prandial blood sugar, all within normal ranges. Nine to 12 individuals in each decade of life were evaluated. Serum GH and Sm-C were measured during waking and sleeping hours; then the effects of exogenous GH were assessed.

In the initial study serum GH was measured throughout 8 waking and 4 sleeping hours and plasma Sm-C was measured at 3:00 PM. A second follow-up study, involving GH administration, lasted 17 days. Subjects ate a constant diet to prepare for the metabolic balance study. The control period lasted 7 days and the treatment period lasted 7 days. During the treatment phase the subjects received 0.168 U GH/kg body weight[3/4] per day at 10:00 AM intramuscularly. Nitrogen, phosphorus, and potassium balance and Sm-C concentration were measured to assess exogenous GH effects.

GH concentrations for 20-29 year olds peaked at 7.3 ng/ml during the day and 20.4 ng/ml during sleep. The average Sm-C level was 1.38 U/ml, and nitrogen, phosphorus, and potassium were all in metabolic balance. Response to GH, in terms of retention of these elements, was slight, and Sm-C levels did not change at all. In 60-79 year olds, however, the average basal Sm-C level was significantly lower than in the younger subjects, 0.62 vs 1.38 U/ml. In six of 12 subjects Sm-C concentration was below the 95 % tolerance limit established by the mean and standard deviation of the younger subjects data (0.64 U/ml lower limit). The subjects with Sm-C > 0.64 U/ml had similar GH secretion patterns to younger subjects and were basically unresponsive to GH treatment in terms of changes in nitrogen, phosphorus, or potassium balance. For these older subjects the mean peak day and night serum GH values were 5.4 and 14.1 ng/ml, respectively, compared to 7.3 and 20.4 in the younger group. In contrast, in the elderly with Sm-C values <0.64 U/ml the peak day and night serum GH concentrations were 3.2 and 3.2 ng/ml. Also, they responded to GH treatment with improved elemental balances, and Sm-C was raised from an initial value of 0.2 U/ml to 0.92 U/ml which was within the normal range for 20-29 year olds. Plasma Sm-C levels declined with age in the 3rd to the 9th decade of life, and nocturnal release of GH correlated closely with Sm-C levels. Age and adiposity accounted for approximately 90 % of the total variability in Sm-C concentration.

In summary:

(1) these data show a progressive decline in GH secretion and plasma Sm-C levels with age,

(2) within each decade of life endogenous GH shows considerable variability,

(3) 55 % of the subjects over age 69 had little day or night release of GH,

(4) this decrease in endogenous GH secretion was associated with an increased anabolic responsiveness to exogenous GH, and

(5) GH decline was also associated with an increase in obesity.

AUTHOR INDEX

Note: Index references to specific bibliographic entries use the citation number for that item when it appears in the text. For example, "4-1" refers to the first entry in Chapter 4. References to terms and concepts in the introduction to a chapter are indicated by the chapter number and "Intro" (e.g., "4-Intro"). Roman numerals refer to a page number in the "Introduction: The Field of Gerontology and the Bibliographies."

SUBJECT INDEX

Note: Index references to specific bibliographic entries use the citation number for that item when it appears in the text. For example, "4-1" refers to the first entry in Chapter 4. References to terms and concepts in the introduction to a chapter are indicated by the chapter number and "Intro" (e.g., "4-Intro"). Roman numerals refer to a page number in the "Introduction: The Field of Gerontology and the Bibliographies."

ABOUT THE EDITOR
AND CONTRIBUTORS

Thomas O. Blank (Ph. D., social psychology, Columbia University), is Associate Professor in the School of Family Studies and Division Director of Social and Behavioral Sciences of the Travelers Center on Aging at the University of Connecticut. He is author of four books and numerous articles on social psychology of aging, housing, and early retirement. Current interests include control processes and dependence in later life, early retirement, and close relationships.

John Contois has a B. S. in biology from University of Massachusetts-- Boston and M. S. in Nutritional Sciences from the University of Connecticut, where he is currently pursuing his doctoral degree, studying diet and lipid metabolism in relation to cardiovascular disease in the elderly. He also was Research Assistant at the USDA Human Nutrition Research Center on Aging at Tufts University.

Mary Ann Kistner, M. A., is a doctoral candidate in the School of Family Studies, University of Connecticut. Her current research is on divorce and midlife women. Other interests include women and aging, identity development across the life-span, intergenerational relationships, non-traditional education, and qualitative research methodology.

Sarah B. Lamm, M. S., received a B.A. in psychology from Purdue University prior to obtaining her M.S. in biobehavioral sciences and Certificate in Gerontology at the University of Connecticut. She then began a research internship at The Ohio Valley Medical Center in Wheeling, West Virginia. She is currently involved in both clinical and research aspects of sleep disorders medicine.

Johanne Philbrick received her Ph. D. in Family Studies with a concentration in gerontology from the University of Connecticut. Her areas of specialization are the history of the science, race and ethnicity among older women, and elderly housing. She lives and works in Connecticut.

Kristin A. Thomas, R. N., M. S., has held various teaching, clinician, and administrative roles in the area of geriatric nursing. She received her B.S.N. from Michigan State University and M.S. (Nursing Administration) and Certificate in Gerontology from the University of Connecticut.

Robert D. Woodcock, M. A., M. Div., M. S. N., is Assistant Professor of Nursing at Western Connecticut State University and a doctoral candidate in Family Studies at the University of Connecticut. He has conducted research in religious studies, community health nursing, and social psychology, most recently examining the roles of family and religious ritual in adapting to later life changes.